HAIRDRESSI

A Salon Ha

HAIRDRESSING DESIGN
A Salon Handbook

Liz Farr

OXFORD
BLACKWELL SCIENTIFIC PUBLICATIONS
LONDON EDINBURGH BOSTON
MELBOURNE PARIS BERLIN VIENNA

Blackwell Scientific Publications
Editorial offices:
Osney Mead, Oxford OX2 0EL
25 John Street, London WC1N 2BL
23 Ainslie Place, Edinburgh EH3 6AJ
3 Cambridge Center, Cambridge,
Massachusetts 02142, USA
54 University Street, Carlton
Victoria 3053, Australia

Other Editorial Offices:
Librairie Arnette SA
2, rue Casimir-Delavigne
75006 Paris
France

Blackwell Wissenschafts-Verlag
Meinekestrasse 4
D-1000 Berlin 15
Germany

Blackwell MZV
Feldgasse 13
A-1238 Wien
Austria

First published 1992

Set by Best-set Typesetter Ltd., Hong Kong
Printed and bound in Great Britain by
Hartnolls, Bodmin, Cornwall

DISTRIBUTORS

Marston Book Services Ltd
PO Box 87
Oxford OX2 0DT
(*Orders*: Tel: 0865 791155
Fax: 0865 791927
Telex: 837515)

USA
Blackwell Scientific Publications, Inc.
3 Cambridge Center
Cambridge, MA 02142
(*Orders*: Tel: 800 759-6102
617 225-0401)

Canada
Oxford University Press
70 Wynford Drive
Don Mills
Ontario M3C 1J9
(*Orders*: Tel: 416 441-2941)

Australia
Blackwell Scientific Publications
(Australia) Pty Ltd
54 University Street
Carlton, Victoria 3053
(*Orders*: Tel: 03 347-0300)

British Library
Cataloguing in Publication Data
Farr, Liz
Hairdressing design.
1. Hairdressing
I. Title
646.7242

ISBN 0-632-02795-9

Library of Congress
Cataloging in Publication Data
Farr, Liz.
Hairdressing design : a salon handbook /
Liz Farr.
p. cm.
Includes index.
ISBN 0-632-02795-9
1. Hairdressing. I. Title.
TT957.F37 1992
646.7′242—dc20

Contents

Introduction vii

1 Basic design 1

1.1 Line 1
1.2 Texture 6
1.3 Shape and proportion 11
1.4 Balance and symmetry 16
1.5 Pattern 18

2 Colour 24

2.1 Colour theory 24
2.2 The colour wheel 27
2.3 Complementary and neutralising colours 27
2.4 Colour terms 30
2.5 Choosing and using colour 31
2.6 Lighting 34
2.7 Questions on colour 34

3 Features influencing hair design 36

3.1 Face shapes 36
3.2 Facial characteristics 43
3.3 The way hair grows 56
3.4 Body characteristics 58
3.5 Image and lifestyle 60
3.6 Questions on features influencing hairdressing design 60

4 **History of fashion and hair styling** 61

4.1 Ancient Egyptians 61
4.2 Ancient Greeks 65
4.3 Ancient Romans 69
4.4 Anglo-Saxons 73
4.5 The Medieval period 74
4.6 15th century and the early Tudor period 83
4.7 Elizabethan period – late 16th century 88
4.8 17th century – the Stuart period 93
4.9 18th century – the Georgian period 98
4.10 19th century 102
4.11 20th century 109
4.12 Fashion trends in the early 1990s 132

5 **Salon design** 138

5.1 Exteriors 138
5.2 Interiors 142

6 **Advertising** 148

6.1 Lay-out 149
6.2 Lettering 150
6.3 Salon advertising 153

7 **Photography** 157

7.1 The camera 158
7.2 Film 160
7.3 Lighting 160
7.4 Composition 161
7.5 Make-up and effects 162
7.6 Personal portfolio 165

8 **The total look** 167

8.1 Different looks from around the world 171
8.2 Developing the total look 178

Index 179

Introduction

Hairdressing is design, whether you are cutting the hair, setting it, colouring it, or perming it. Hairdressers use their creative ability alongside their technical skill to offer a creative service to the client. Hairdressers may not be aware at the time of all the design decisions they are making. As with the artist at the canvas the decisions come intuitively, because they feel right, but before this stage can be achieved the hairdresser, like the artist, must be trained in the basic language of design. Only then can they draw upon this wealth of information and adapt it to an appropriate situation. The hairdresser should feel confident in being able to cope with whatever walks through the salon door (from my experience with only a *few* exceptions!), whether it is the older client who wants a tight perm or a set, or the younger client who wants the latest cut, colour or half-shaven head. This is why it is important that stylists have a good understanding of design so that they really *know* what they are doing and can project a real sense of confidence in their clients.

Hairdressing training is an important part of a stylist's career and is a formative part of professional development. This initial training should include a good basic design element and also provide lots of opportunity for the simultaneous development of creative ability and technical skill as well as offering every possible opportunity and encouragement to exhibit these combined skills.

In order to be adaptable, it is important that the hairdresser should be able to expand on technical skill to offer a complete service to the client and indeed work in tandem with the other fashion areas that are involved in creating the total image. This is the only way we will be able to gain full recognition and demonstrate that hairdressers are in fact creative designers. In order to compete in this ever-changing fashion world, hairdressers must, firstly, keep abreast of current fashion trends (whether they happen to like them or not) as hairdressing is a vital part of the fashion image. Secondly, hairdressers must be able not only to adapt to new ideas but also to be the innovators of new ideas and techniques themselves. It stands to reason that if they ignore the world around them then the world will undoubtedly ignore them too, and the possibilities of attracting new customers and expanding businesses will be minimal.

This book aims to identify and simplify the basic principles of design that are involved in hairdressing. It will assist hairdressers in identifying those principles, understanding them and indeed applying them to practical situations, in order to enhance the hairdressers' professional development and last but certainly not least their salon performance and credibility.

1

Basic Design

Basic design may not seem initially important or obviously relevant to the novice hairdresser, but as in any creative profession basic design is the essential background ingredient for a true awareness of line, shape, texture, proportion, balance and pattern creation. This extends into every creative task the hairdresser encounters, including hair analysis, cutting, blow-drying, setting, etc., so that once the hairdresser has acquired an understanding of these basics in design, they can be used as a springboard for many inspiring ideas and innovative creations.

It is sometimes difficult for novice hairdressers when striving to gain an understanding of basic design not to become blinkered into only accepting things that seem directly relevant to hairdressing. They need to remind themselves that sometimes by treading further afield and accepting other information from disciplines outside hairdressing they can acquire a wider scope of knowledge which, if they allow it, will enhance their personal development and creative vocabulary.

1.1 LINE

Line is the fundamental language used in basic design. It can be used in numerous ways to convey visual information and can be very versatile in its appearance to create many different effects.

When you draw lines they usually take on a direction that indicates their character. They might rise or fall, flow or appear hesitant, and they can be expressive as shown in Fig. 1.1.

If there is more than one line then again the way in which they are drawn in relation to each other indicates their overall character (Fig. 1.2). They might collide and crisscross giving the appearance of disorder, or they might be regimented, giving the appearance of control and regulation. Figure 1.3

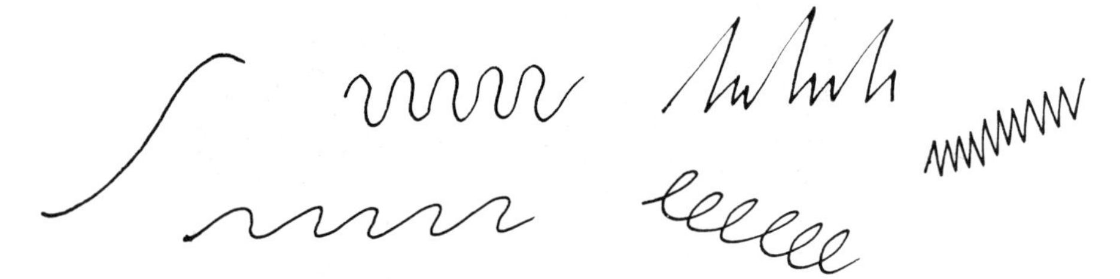

Fig. 1.1 Character of a single line.

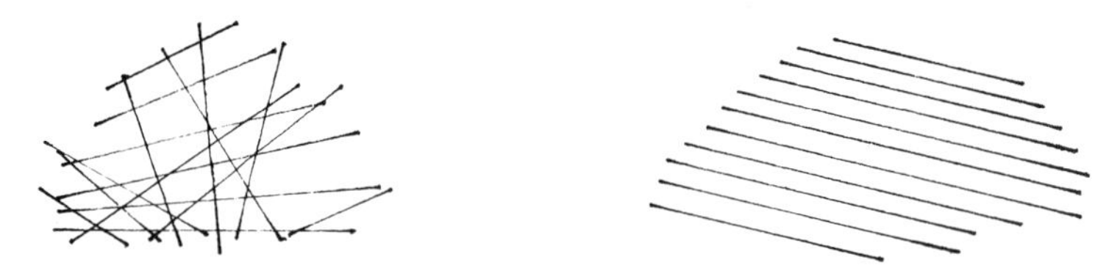

Fig. 1.2 Overall character of lines.

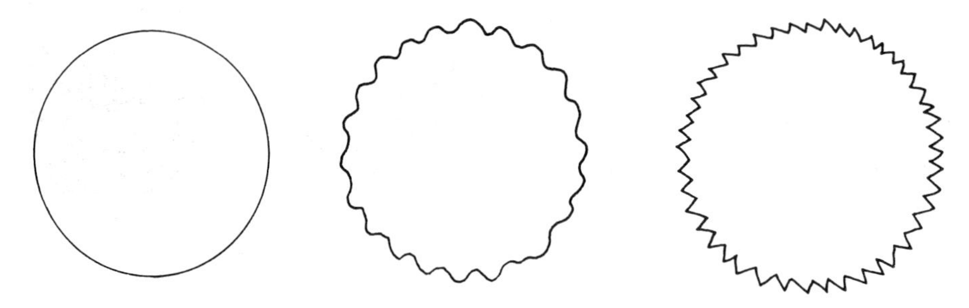

Fig. 1.3 Line suggesting surface quality.

shows outline being used to suggest a solid form. The type of line used will determine the quality of the object's surface, e.g. smooth, wavy, spiky.

Line can be extremely versatile when illustrating information or ideas, especially if different media are used. A line drawn with a 2H pencil will appear totally different and suggest a different image to a line drawn with a crayon. Its surface quality will give it a textural appearance. This is worth knowing when certain effects are needed. For instance, if you wanted to suggest a wavy head of hair, it would probably be easiest and most effective to use a crayon, pen and ink or paint to lend a flow to the hair. On the other hand, if you wanted to draw a sharp, geometric cut it would be best to use pencil or pen to give more control over the line. It will help you when you want to illustrate a certain type of hair style or texture to know which is the best selection of lines to employ.

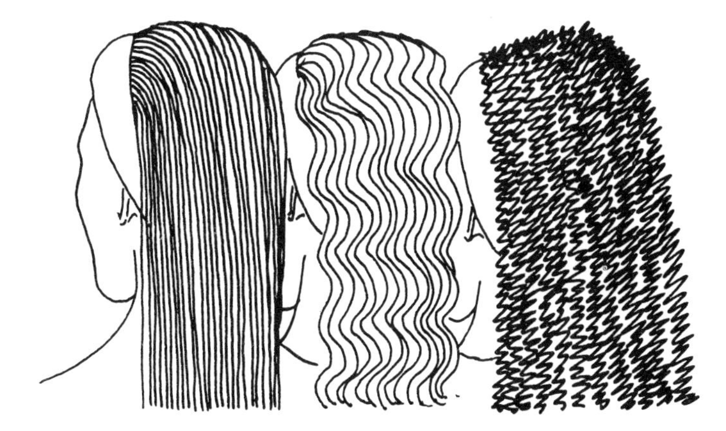

Fig. 1.4 Line represents different hair types.

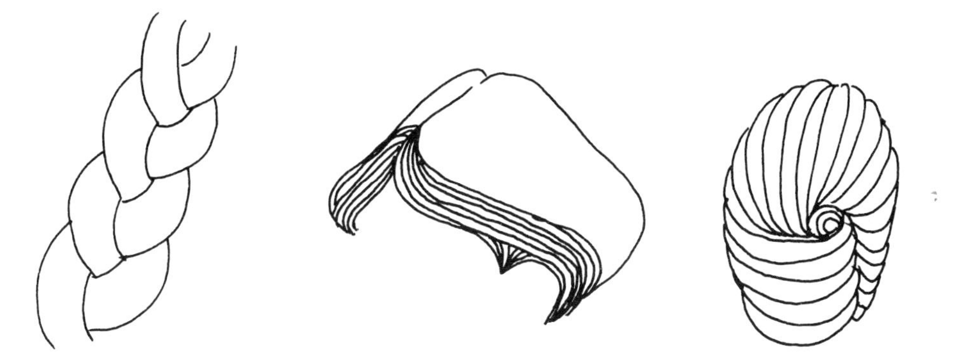

Fig. 1.5 Line used to demonstrate basic form.

How is line used in hairdressing?

In hairdressing it is easy to think of hair as a mass of lines, whether straight, wavy, curly or frizzy. These might be regular lines that are formed into a pattern, such as an S shape in waved hair, or irregular lines that are not in a formulated pattern, such as in frizzy hair. Some examples are shown in Fig. 1.4. Or line can be used in hairdressing to demonstrate basic forms, as shown in Fig. 1.5, or to suggest different textures as shown in Fig. 1.6.

Line is important in hairdressing for three specific reasons:

(1) It helps us to identify shape (Fig. 1.7).
(2) We need to have a good vocabulary of different line variations when we want to communicate ideas or receive information (Fig. 1.8).
(3) It dictates the overall *shape* of objects or, for our purpose, hair. The

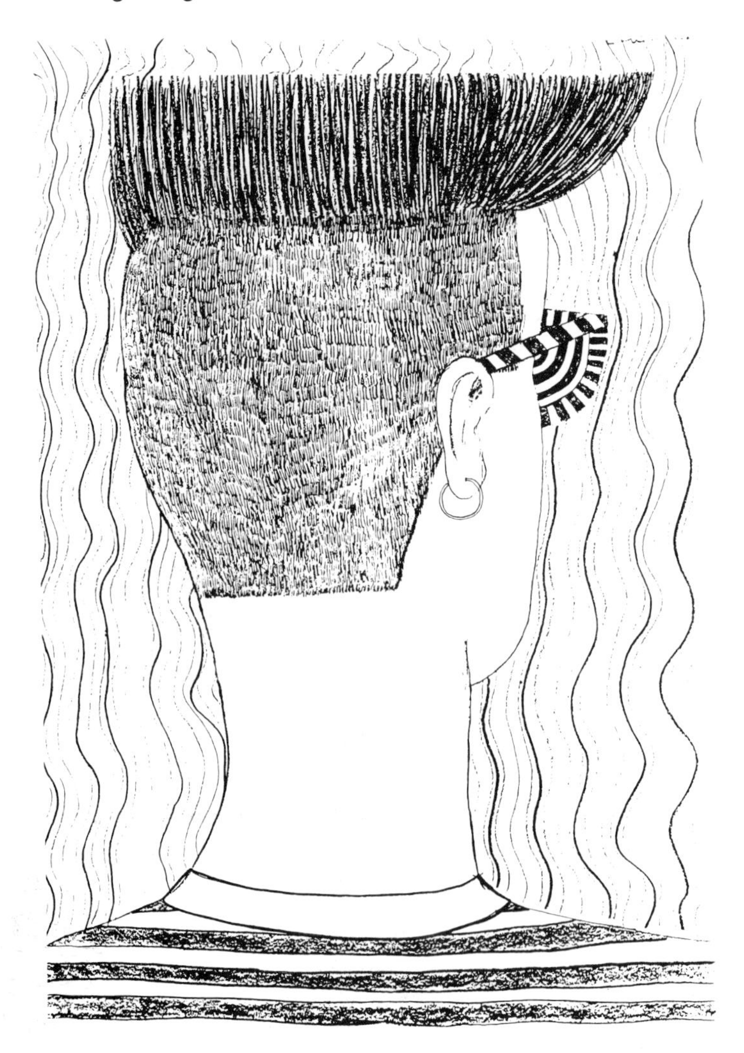

Fig. 1.6 Example of a student's work showing the use of different lines to suggest different textures.

overall line of a hair style will carry the eye of the viewer and determine its total shape (Fig. 1.9a).

Using line to identify shape is equally important to the hairdresser when cutting the hair. For instance, the line of a layered cut, where the hair is held out and cut at a 90 degree angle from the head, follows the contour of the head and takes on a rounded shape. A long layered or graduated cut, on the other hand, has different lengths of hair blended together by altering the angle between 45 degrees and 180 degrees and will result overall in a diamond shape. A one-length cut, where the weight and fullness of the cut is around the perimeter of the hair, will result in a triangular shape (Fig. 1.9b).

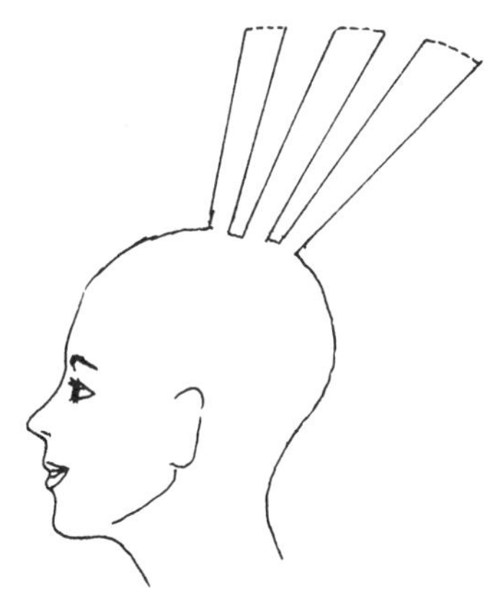

Fig. 1.7 Line used to define shape.

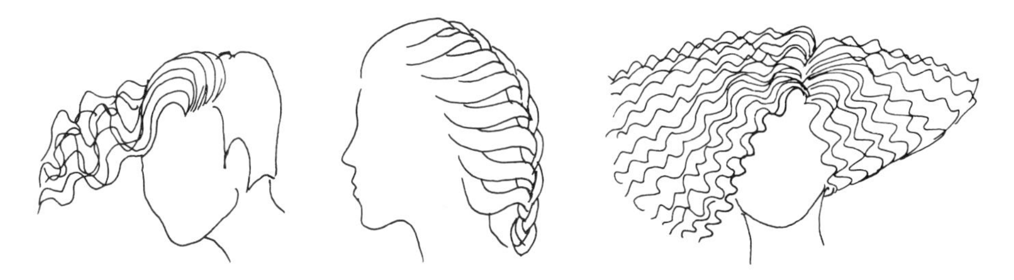

Fig. 1.8 Line variations used to communicate ideas.

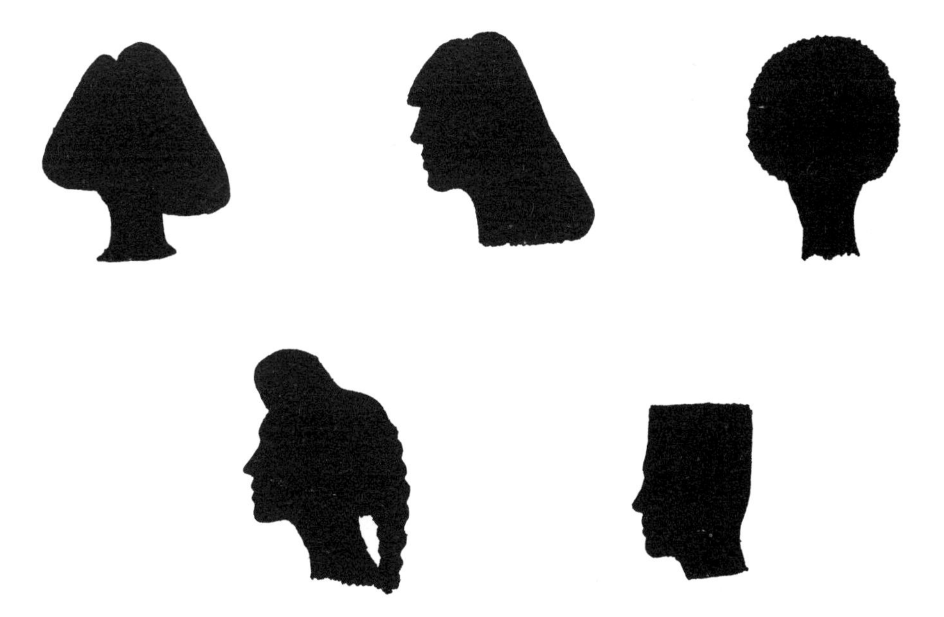

Fig. 1.9a The overall line of a hair style, shown in the silhouettes, defines the total shape.

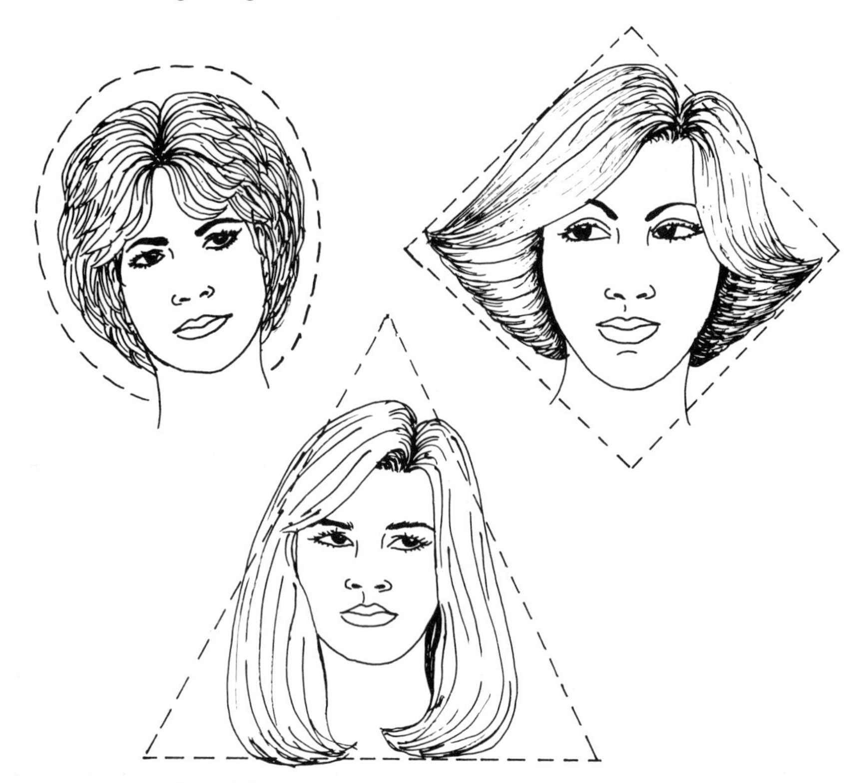

Fig. 1.9b Basic cutting lines and overall shapes.

1.2 TEXTURE

To be able to recognise different textures is an extremely important attribute for any hair stylist. The type and texture of the hair can determine what style is worn successfully. When a client comes into the salon the stylist should know at a glance if the hair style the client requires is suitable to that particular hair texture. If any processes, such as perming or straightening the hair, have to be used in order to achieve the style, then the following factors must be borne in mind:

(1) Is the client's hair texture suitable for the process to be used?
(2) Will the client be able to cope with this new 'textured' hair?

Most people learn the limitations of their hair with the help and advice of their hairdresser, so when a client comes into the salon for a slinky fashionable bob, and her hair texture is incompatible, be honest but constructive in your advice. Don't just inform her that her hair won't go like that, but instead offer her something that would suit her, her hair texture and her face shape, and something that she will find easy to manage.

The stylist might have the skill to scrunch dry body perms or straighten the hair with blow drying, but it is necessary to determine whether or not the client has the skills to cope with her own hair in this way. Although the client may be delighted with the results in the salon, the success of your creation also depends strongly on the after care.

In order to be able to identify the variations of texture, let us look at what it actually is.

What is texture?

Texture usually describes the sensation we experience from the surface of an object or substance. The ability to recognise different textures and their limitations is something that has to be learned mostly through experience, but a basic understanding of what happens when we see or feel a texture will help explain its properties.

Firstly, when we are confronted with a texture it arouses two of our senses:

(1) *Touch*. Our fingers help to identify the properties of a texture, e.g. smooth, harsh, spiky. Even though we might not be able to see the texture our touching fingers stimulate the memory automatically to provide a sensory reaction or sensation that identifies the textural qualities.

How often have you found your way along in the dark by feeling; being able to recognise and identify different surfaces by just touching them? Or do you dislike a certain food because the texture does not feel pleasant in the mouth.

(2) *Sight*. Although unaccompanied by our fingers, our eyes scan different textures, for instance when looking through a magazine, and our memory identifies the different textural qualities that are compatible with what we see.

You only have to look at magazines or newspapers to see a whole array of different surface textures that arouse your sense of touch, from photographs of food and fabrics to surfaces, such as wood and stone. Looking at different hair textures should arouse the same sensory reactions. When a client comes into the salon, first your eyes scan the hair, trying to identify its texture, then when you get to touch the hair the fingers usually confirm your predictions.

Hair types and textures

Variation in hair types and textures reflects the physical characteristics that exist in different races (Fig. 1.10) and this is an important feature to recognise and respect:

(1) *Afro hair* types are usually curly and their texture usually fine. The hair

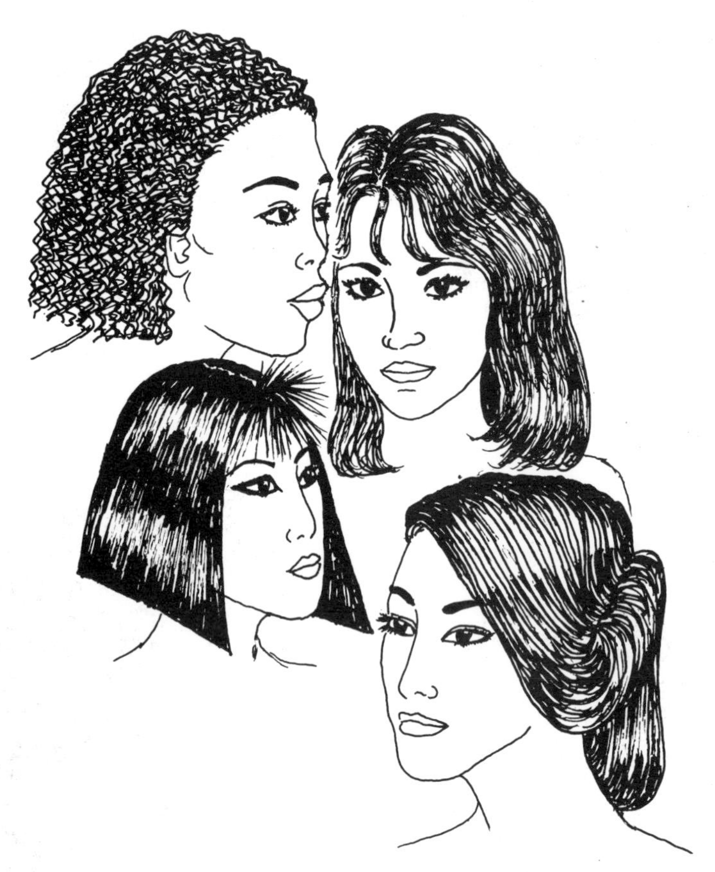

Fig. 1.10 Hair types characteristic of different races.

is quite dry and fragile and it needs a lot of care and attention. It is mostly dark brown or occasionally black in colour, due to the increased amounts of melanin present, which protects against the sun.

(2) *Asian and Oriental hair* types are usually straight and the texture is thick. The hair is usually very strong and has a tendency to resist chemical processes. The colour is dark brown or black, and occasionally the black tends to have a bluish tone to it.

(3) *European hair* varies immensely in type, texture and colour. The hair type ranges between straight, kinky, wavy and curly and the texture might be anything from fine to coarse. It tends to be of medium strength and usually accepts chemical processes. The colour can vary from blonde to red through to dark brown, but is very rarely black. There is less melanin in European hair so it is not so well protected against strong sunlight.

Hair types

There are six basic hair types:

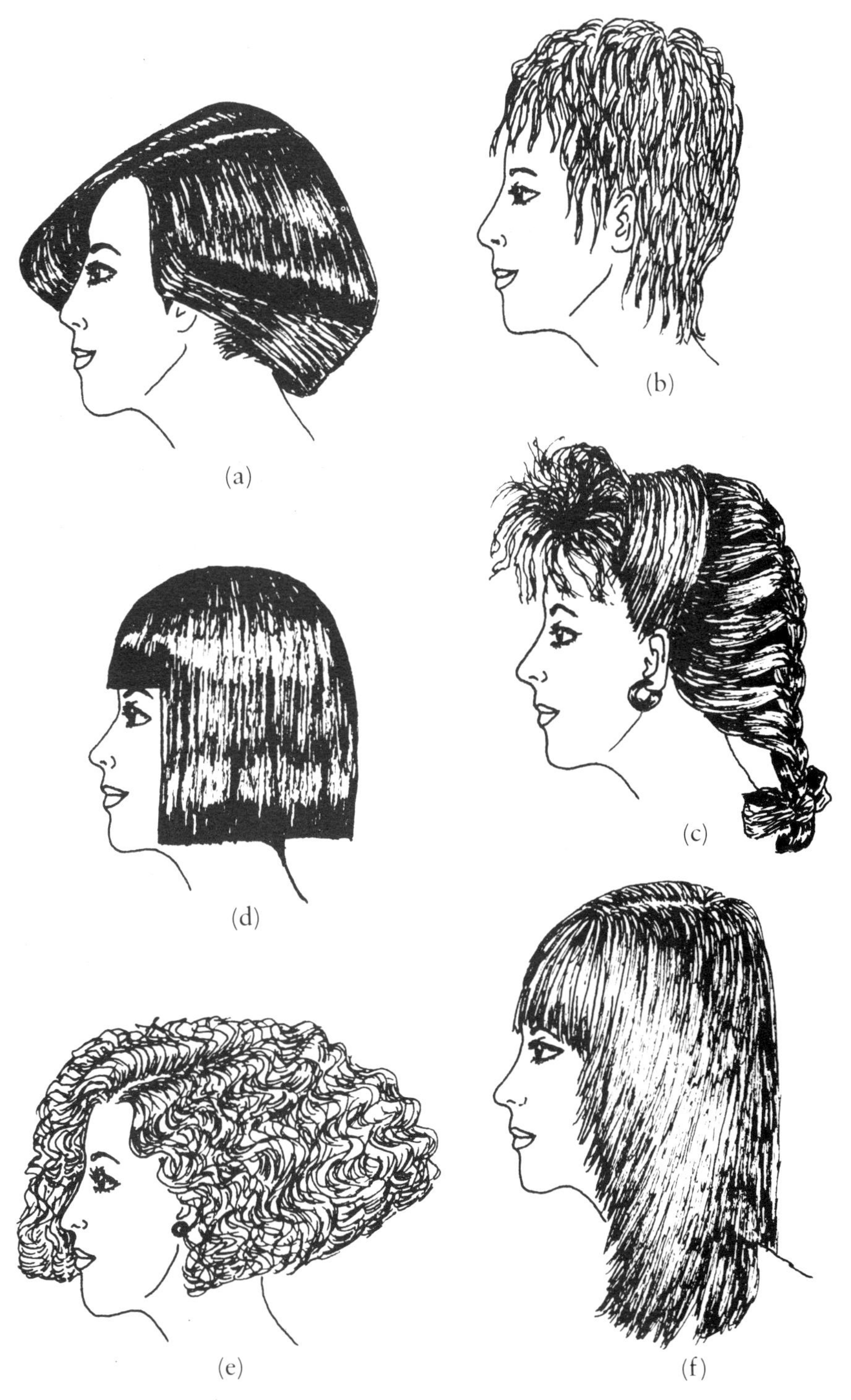

Fig. 1.11 Hair styles that are compatible with the six different hair types: (a) thick; (b) thin; (c) coarse; (d) straight; (e) curly; (f) fine.

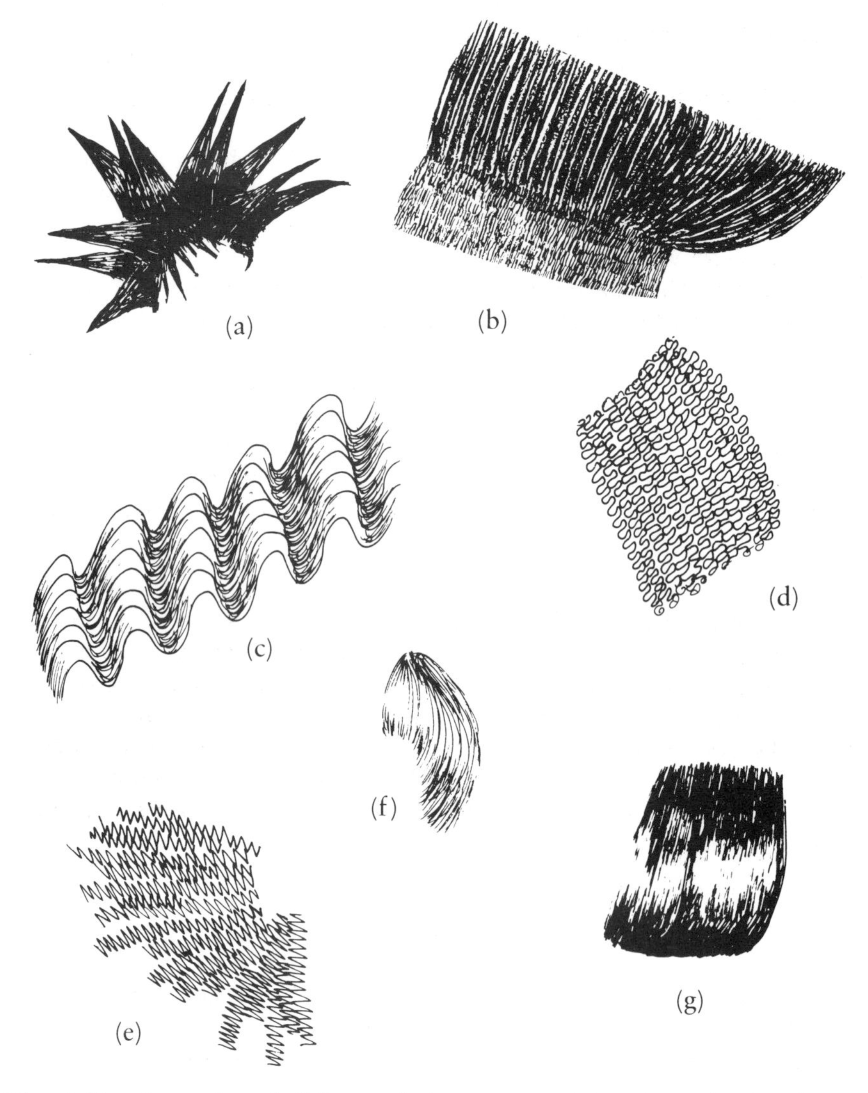

Fig. 1.12 Examples of different hair textures: (a) spikey; (b) bristly; (c) wavy; (d) curly; (e) frizzy; (f) soft; (g) smooth.

(1) *Thin hair*. The actual diameter of each hair is narrow, and so the effect tends to look sparse. The hair is soft and silky so it needs careful handling. Precision cutting is required to give shape, and perming, if suitable, to give body and style.
(2) *Fine hair*. Although each hair is narrow in diameter there is plenty of hair. It still needs careful handling because it tends to be fly-away and can be difficult to control. One of the common features of this type is that it can be difficult to perm and is usually best kept short or in long layers.

(3) *Thick hair.* The diameter of each hair is wide, so the hair tends to be heavy. There is usually quite a lot of hair and it can be difficult to handle. It is best kept under control by wearing it in shorter graduation or bob-type cuts.
(4) *Coarse hair.* This hair feels harsh to touch and tends not to shine very much. It usually appears abundant with the outer layers sometimes looking quite frizzy. The hair lacks elasticity and so does not hold a set or blow-dry very well.
(5) *Curly hair.* This hair has natural elasticity and curl. It can be worn any length, except that wearing it long tends to straighten the curl slightly so it can become wavy. Layering will increase the curl. This hair is quite easy to manage. Depending on the degree of curl, it can also be straightened with the use of larger rollers or by blow-drying.
(6) *Straight hair.* This type has no natural movement whatsoever. It can be difficult to manage, and certainly difficult to curl or perm. Sets or blow-dries tend to drop easily. It is best cut into a style such as a bob.

Hair texture

The words we use to describe particular textures, e.g. soft, sticky, pitted, brittle, hard, fluffy, all conjure up images of a surface or object. The language we use to distinguish hair textures describes to us what we expect to feel when we touch it, e.g. spiky, frizzy, smooth, prickly, soft, curly, wavy.

Once the skill of being able to identify the combination of hair types and hair textures is gained, the hairdresser will be able to offer invaluable advice about suitable hair styles for particular types and textures. Some examples are shown in Figs. 1.11 and 1.12.

Exercises in identifying texture

Hairdressing trainees in colleges and salons can help themselves to identify different textures and to clarify hair types and hair textures in their minds by collecting photographs from magazines. A catalogue could be made up with a page or two for each texture, showing also suitable styles for the various textures. There could also be some pages for different hair types, including suitable styles for each type too.

1.3 SHAPE AND PROPORTION

Being unable to draw, in particular the face, is one of the biggest setbacks hairdressing students seem to have, and yet to be able to quickly jot down ideas and styles would clearly help them communicate better with clients. The problem seems to be that sometime in their distant past someone has told them that they cannot draw and this assumption has become a deep-rooted fact which creates a barrier that is extremely difficult to penetrate. Many a good idea has been crushed because of this. Drawing is an individual

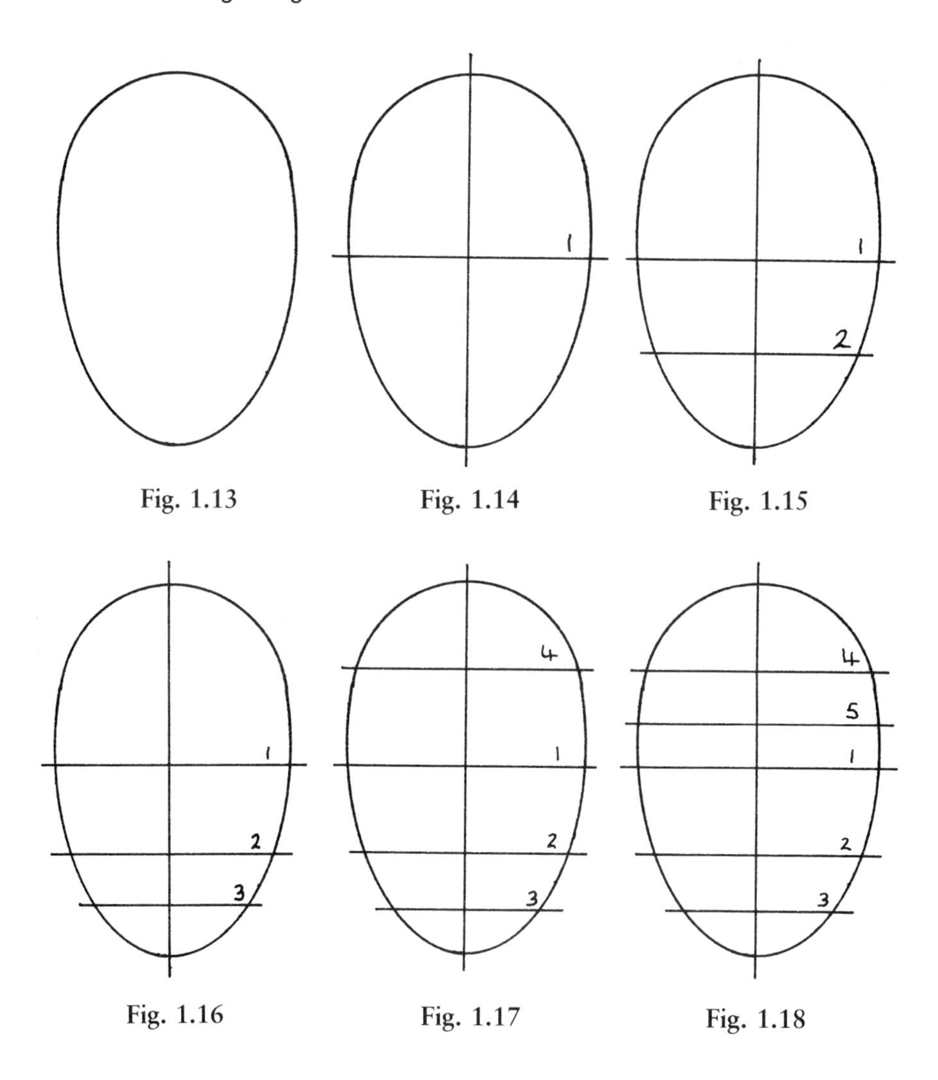

Fig. 1.13 Fig. 1.14 Fig. 1.15

Fig. 1.16 Fig. 1.17 Fig. 1.18

form of expression and there should be no strict standards, good or bad, to it. Maybe sometimes students have been led to believe that a drawing has to be realistic to be good and that if you do not have the skill to draw realistically then you cannot draw. This is absurd. The key to being able to draw is the combination of developing the ability to observe and put down on paper what you see and having a good knowledge of the tools and materials and their possibilities.

Drawing a face

Drawing a face can be done through following a simple set of steps that chart out the proportions of the face, and tips on drawing the features. There are different technical methods of drawing a face and head, although they do seem to depend on quite a lot of measuring. For our purpose a simple basic method that acts as a good rough guide in simply plotting the basic proportions is all we require.

Basic proportions – step-by-step

(1) *Fig. 1.13*. Draw a rough oval shape, so it resembles an egg, slightly wider at the top and narrower at the bottom.
(2) *Fig. 1.14*. Draw a horizontal line straight through the centre of this oval shape. (Call this line 1: it will indicate the position of the eyes.). Then draw a vertical line that also cuts through the centre.
(3) *Fig. 1.15*. Half way between your first horizontal line and the bottom of the oval draw a second horizontal line. (Call this line 2: it will indicate the tip of the nose.)
(4) *Fig. 1.16*. Draw in a third horizontal line between the last horizontal line and the bottom of the oval. (Call this line 3: it will indicate the position of the lips.)
(5) *Fig. 1.17*. Go back to line 1 and now draw another horizontal line half way up to the top of the oval. (Call this line 4: it will indicate the position of the hairline.)
(6) *Fig. 1.18*. The last horizontal line should now be drawn half way between line 1 and line 4. (Call this line 5: it will indicate the position of the eyebrows.)

Plotting the features

The basic positions of the features are now in place. The eyes should be positioned evenly on line 1 and the size of each eye should allow an imaginary third eye to sit comfortably between them. Also note that eyes are usually almond shaped and have sockets, lids and an iris that spans from the top lid to the bottom lid and also eyelashes. Eyebrows usually span the width of the eye, starting above the inside corner of the eye and finishing at the outside corner of the eye.

The nose sits straight down the vertical line in the centre of the face. The width of the base of the nose is usually the same width as the space between the eyes.

The lips sit centrally on the line and if you took an imaginary vertical line from the centre of each eye down to the lips this will indicate where they usually finish.

Ears sit on the sides of the face and the top sits on the eye line and the bottom sits on the nose line.

The top of the oval indicates the top of the head, so when you are drawing hair styles the hair should start from the hairline (line 4).

The position of the neck starts at the base of the jaw line and tends to curve in slightly when viewed from the front (Figs 1.19 and 1.20.)

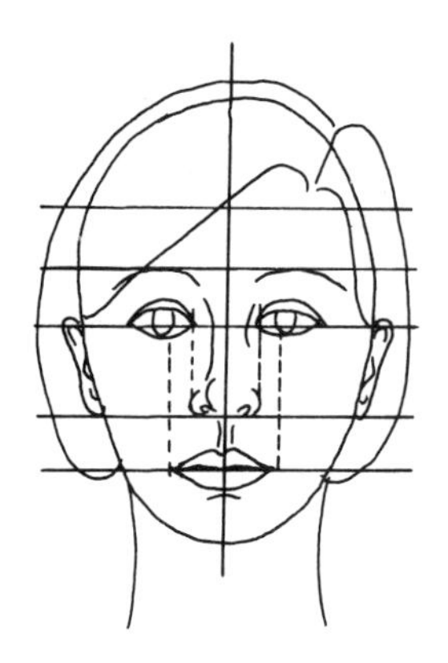

Fig. 1.19 Plotting the features.

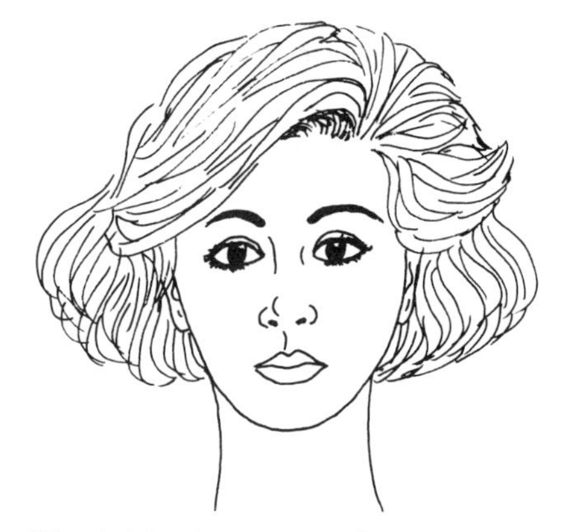

Fig. 1.20 Drawing a face – the finished look.

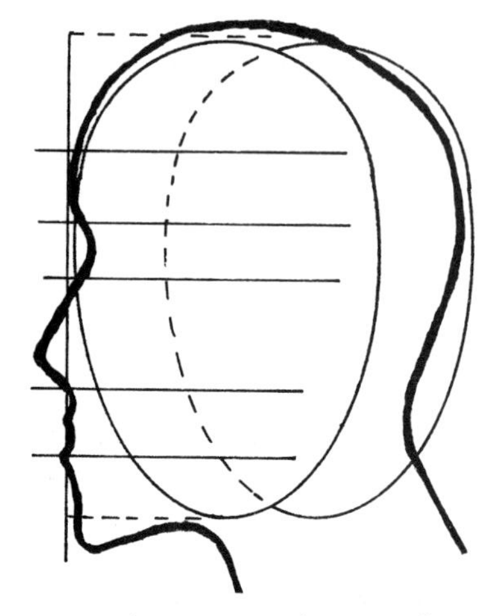

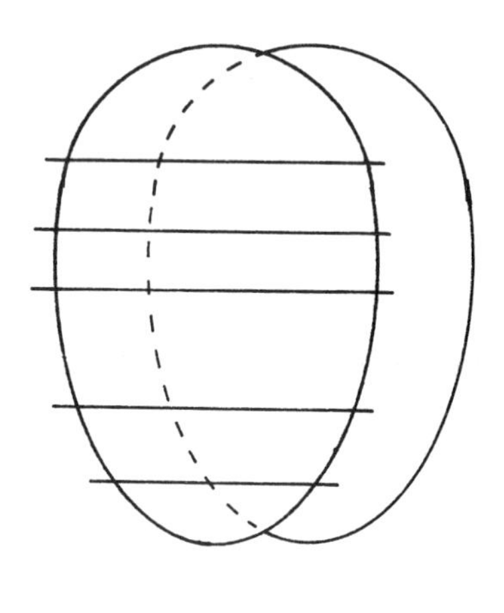

Fig. 1.21 Adapting the same proportions to draw a profile.

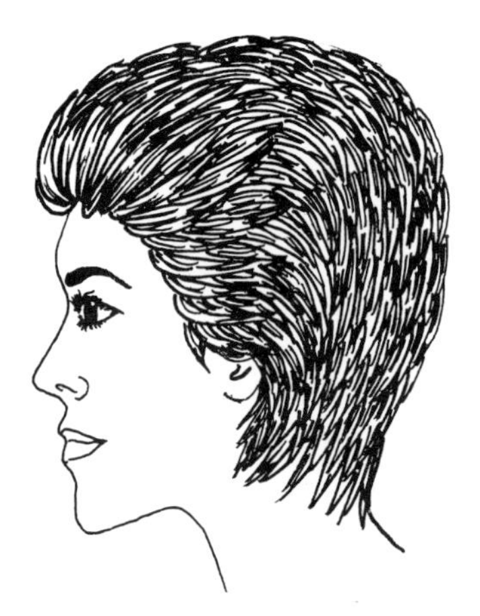

Fig. 1.22 The finished profile.

Drawing a profile

The simple method described above can also be applied to drawing a profile, but you have to remember you are only seeing half of the features (unless of course you are into Cubism like Picasso!). The positions are the same. The only difference is that your vertical line should have moved to the outside of one of the edges of the basic oval shape, and that the eyebrow line, lips and chin will all meet this vertical line. The nose will protrude over it. The width of the head in profile is also important; it is always bigger than you imagine. If you draw a second oval shape over the top of the first but move it to one side about a quarter of the width of the oval, this will indicate the width of the skull (Figs. 1.21 and 1.22).

Figure drawing

It might be helpful to you also to know a simple method of plotting down the proportions of a figure. Basically the head should fit into the body six or seven times, although fashion illustrators tend to lengthen that proportion because it is more flattering. The head should fit in twice to the width of the shoulders (Fig. 1.23).

Drawing by the grid method

Another method of drawing that can be extremely useful and guarantees accuracy is using a grid. This method also allows you to enlarge or reduce the image.

Copying an image using the grid method – step by step (Figs 1.24 and 1.25)

(1) Choose a photograph from a magazine of a well-defined portrait of a male or female with an interesting hair style.

(2) Divide the photograph up into a grid of small squares (depending on the size of the picture: the bigger the picture the bigger the squares you need to use). To make 2 cm squares, for example, use a ruler to make marks every 2 cm round all sides of the picture. When you have done this, join the dots with a ruler to make straight lines across and down the picture. Finally, number your grid of squares across the top and down the left hand side.

(3) Using a pencil, draw an identical grid of squares and number it in the same way. (To enlarge your drawing, you would use larger squares, e.g. 2 cm squares would become 4 cm squares, or if you wanted to reduce the drawing you would use smaller squares, e.g. 2 cm squares would become 1 cm squares.)

(4) Once you have drawn the grid, then start to copy the photographic

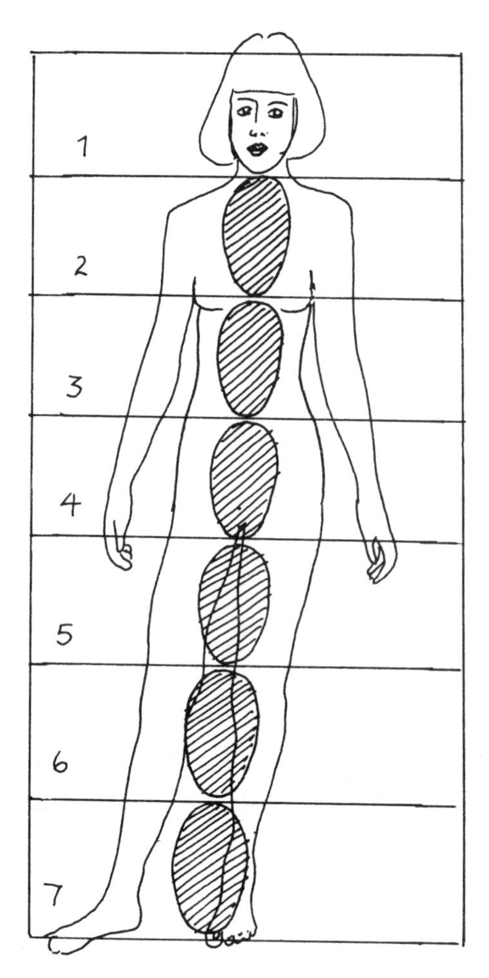

Fig. 1.23 The proportions of figure drawing.

image onto your paper by taking one square at a time and drawing exactly what you see in each corresponding square, checking all the time by cross reference. Treat it like a large jig-saw and you are making the picture up square by square.

(5) When you have completed the drawing and it is accurate, then finish by carefully rubbing out your grid.

1.4 BALANCE AND SYMMETRY

To be able to understand balance and apply that understanding is extremely important to hairdressers. They need not only the ability to differentiate between balanced and unbalanced styles, but also to be able to demonstrate their knowledge and skill in balancing clients' facial and body features with

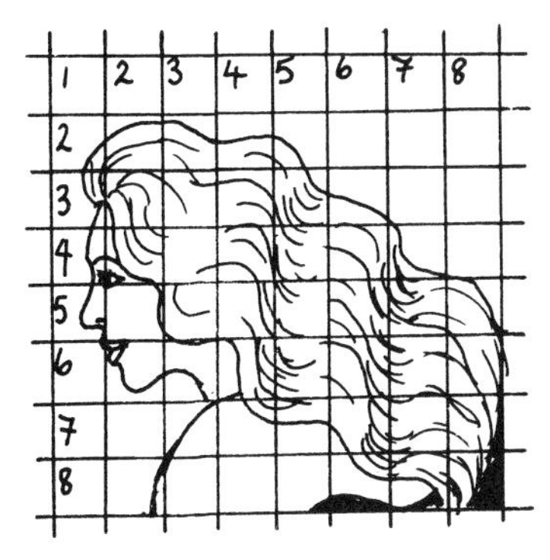

Fig. 1.24 Drawing by the grid method: 5 mm squares.

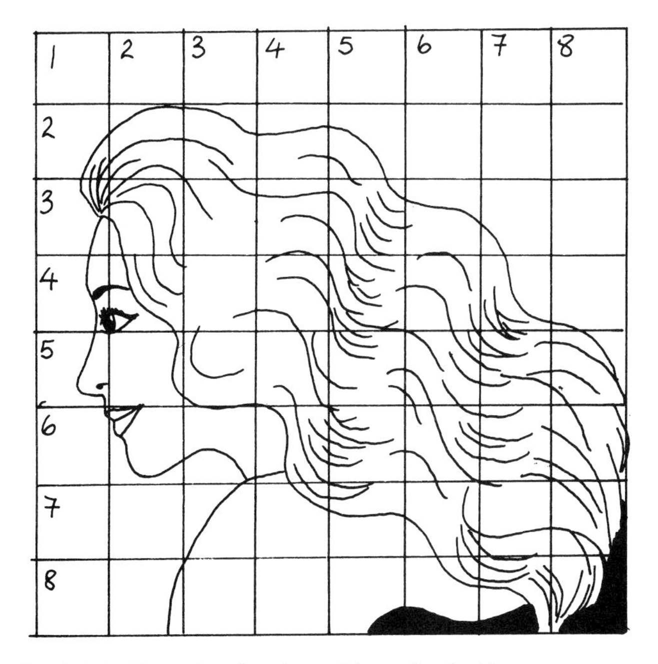

Fig. 1.25 Drawing by the grid method: 10 mm squares.

suitable hair styles, and offering sound advice on unsuitable styles to avoid. It is natural for the human eye to seek symmetry and balance in line, on a plane or in objects. The ancient Egyptians and Greeks were the masters of creating symmetry and it applied to everything, including their hair styles. Since then it has played a major part in hair styling throughout time, as we can see in Chapter 4 – History of Fashion and Hair Styling.

Balance and symmetry basically mean the same thing in hairdressing – that is the exact correspondence of parts on either side of a straight line or plane, equal or in harmony. A hair style that is equally proportioned on the head and with one side corresponding to the other is well-balanced and

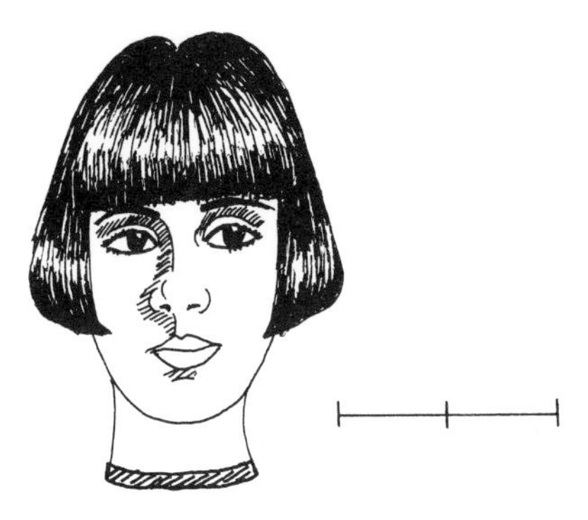

Fig. 1.26 An evenly balanced symmetrical style.

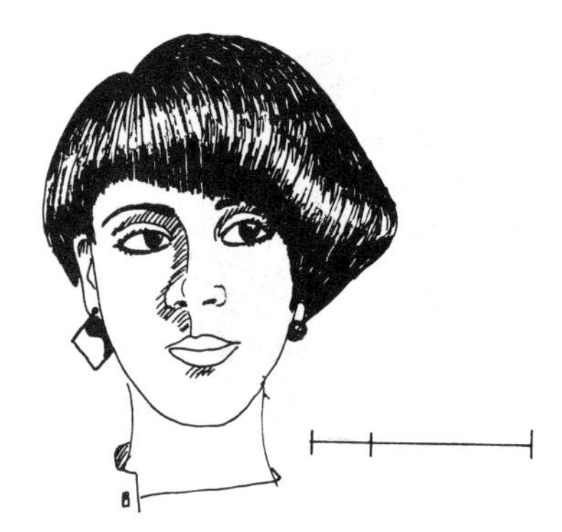

Fig. 1.27 An unbalanced asymmetrical style.

symmetrical. For example, a straightforward short bob is a symmetrical hair style (Fig. 1.26).

Unbalanced styling or asymmetry is the opposite. It is out of proportion and in want of symmetry. The hair is not equally proportioned on the head, and one side does not necessarily correspond to the other side. For example, in the 1960s the asymmetric bob was a popular hair style which consisted of the hair being cut in an unbalanced way, with one side shorter than the other (Fig. 1.27). Figure 1.28 shows some examples of symmetrical and asymmetrical hair styles.

1.5 PATTERN

Although shape and proportion are important to the hairdresser, so too are the possibilities of pattern. An awareness of potential patterns can help inspire creative ideas and many patterns can be adapted into hair designs. We have already mentioned that the eye automatically seeks symmetry in whatever it sees and the same principle applies to pattern. A pattern looks appealing because it achieves balance as well as looking interesting.

In order to distinguish pattern possibilities let us look at the basic principles of actually creating patterns. Patterns are built up from separate units (shapes or lines) which are arranged in some form of repeat. This repeated motif is then formatted into a network or grid for pattern making, and the way this is done can vary. For a regular repeated pattern the lines or shapes are repeated on a *block repeat* (Fig. 1.29). For a variation it can fit into a *half-drop repeat* (Fig. 1.30) or a *diamond repeat* (Fig. 1.31).

Although patterns are usually determined by the network or grid employed, further variations can be introduced by actually rotating the shapes themselves inside the network or grid by, for example, 360 degrees or 180 degrees, or even by reversing them. So, as we can see in Fig. 1.32, the possibilities of pattern from one shape or source are enormous.

Of course other methods of pattern creation can be employed, for instance,

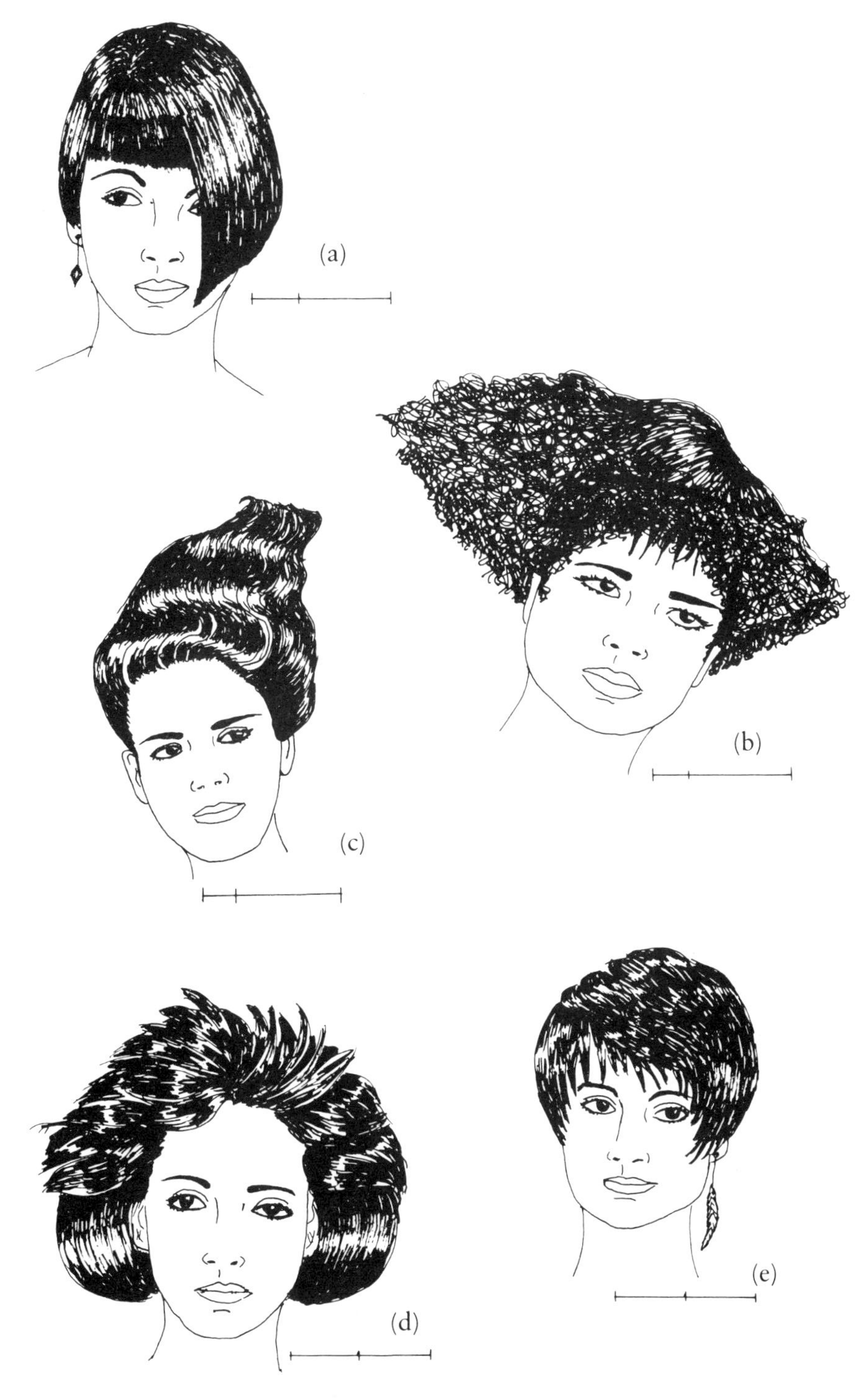

Fig. 1.28 Symmetrical and asymmetrical styles: (a), (b) and (c) are asymmetrical; (d) and (e) are symmetrical.

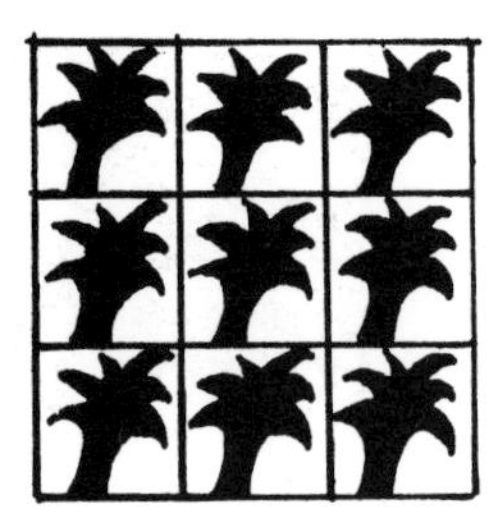

Fig. 1.29 Block repeat grid.

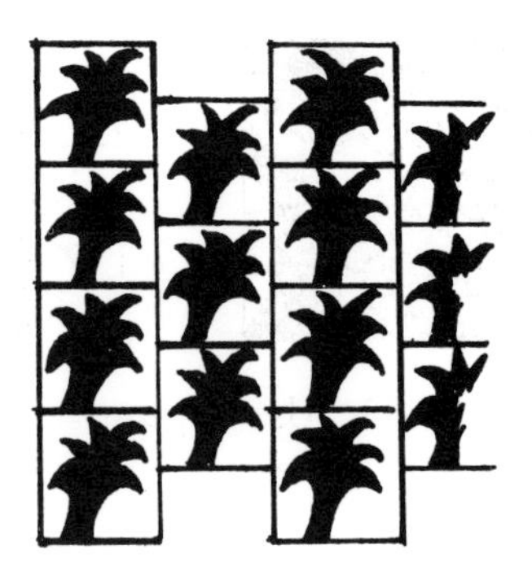

Fig. 1.30 Half drop repeat.

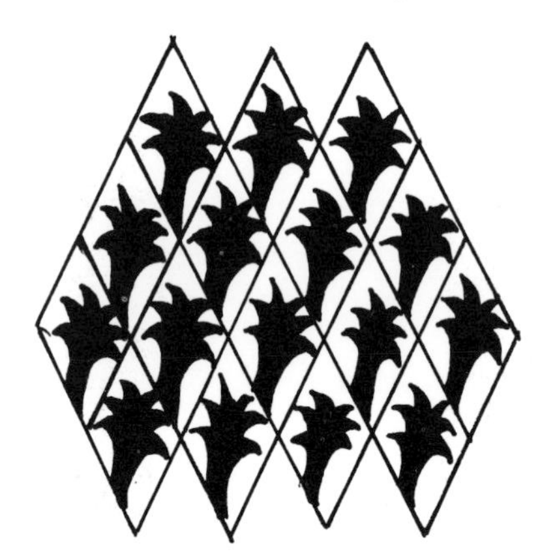

Fig. 1.31 Diamond repeat.

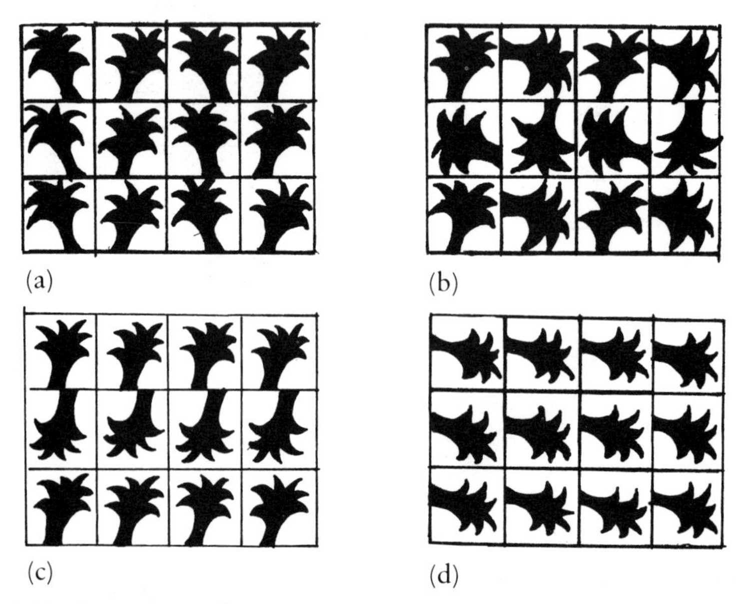

Fig. 1.32 Variations of pattern within the grid: (a) reverse repeat; (b) 360° rotation; (c) 180° rotation; (d) 90° rotation.

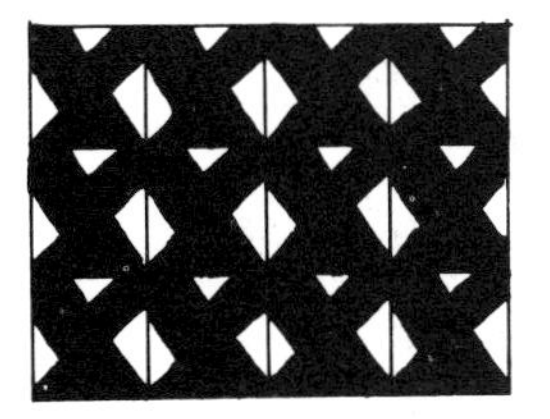
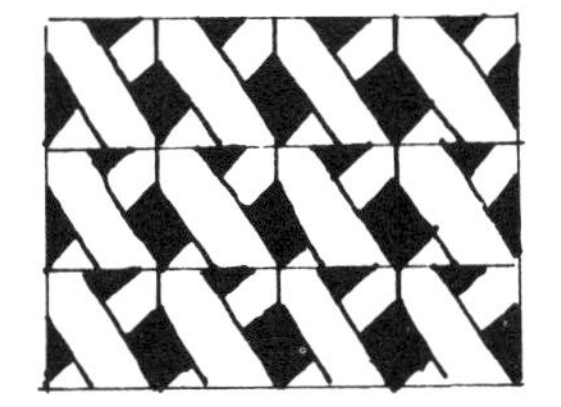
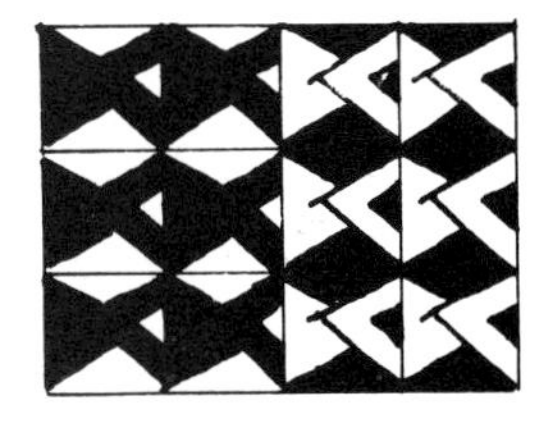

Fig. 1.33 Use of positive and negative shapes to make patterns.

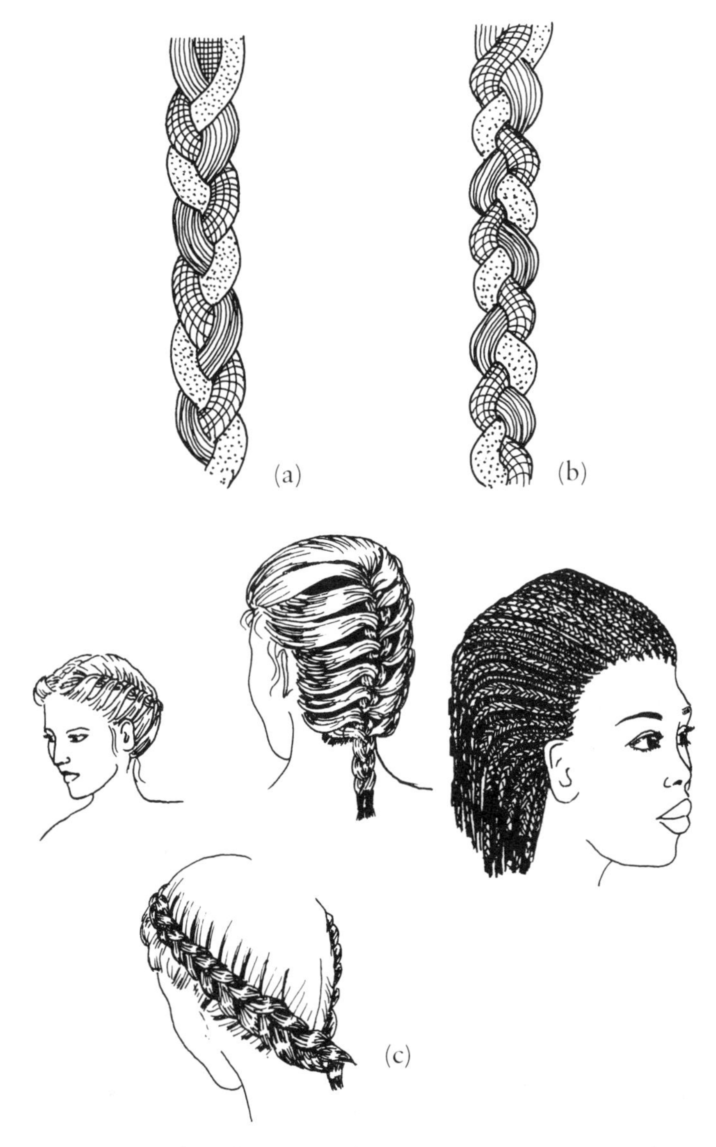

Fig. 1.34 Example of a three-strand plait: (a) strands passed over each other; (b) strands passed under each other; (c) different effects.

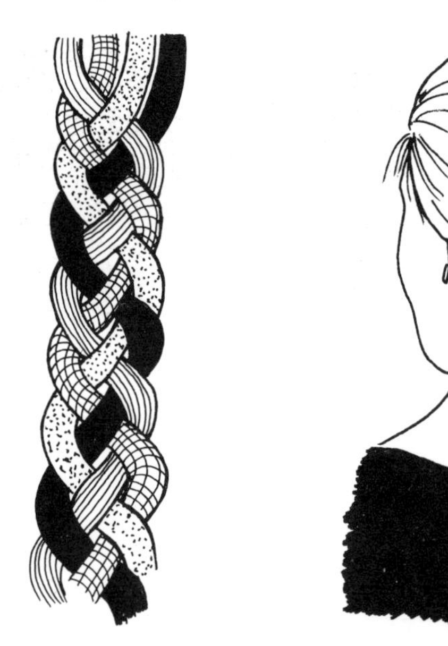

Fig. 1.35 Four-stem braid.

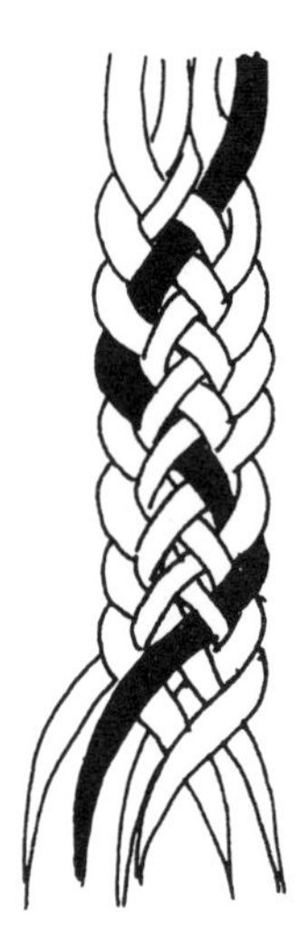

Fig. 1.36 Six-strand plait.

by looking at positive and negative shapes. The variations on this again can be infinite (Fig. 1.33).

Pattern in hairdressing design

The most common form of pattern creation in hairdressing is by use of the *plait*. Different variations of plaiting have become very popular over the last

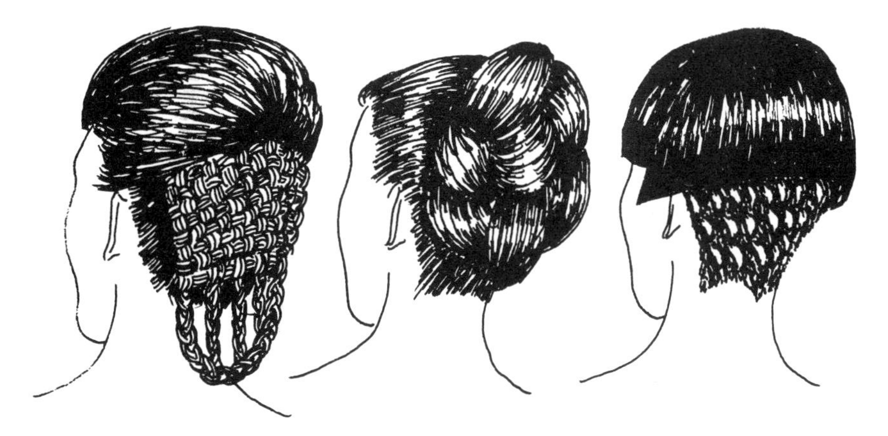

Fig. 1.37 Pattern used in hair styling.

20 years, especially from the strong African influence of the 1970s. Tribal plaiting has inspired many creations in Western styles for both black and white people. Here are some examples:

Three-strand plait. This can be woven by passing strands of hair over the top of each other or alternatively underneath each other. This plait is employed in 'French plaiting' or 'corn rowing' (Fig. 1.34).

Four-stem braid. This makes an interesting pattern and can be worn as a flat plait (Fig. 1.35).

Six-strand plait. A plait using six strands takes more skill but can give a very woven effect (Fig. 1.36).

Other patterns besides plaiting can be designed into the hair style. Long hair, for instance, is a good medium for experimenting on possibilities. Another example is the trend of actually cutting particular patterns or images into the shorn head, so that the head becomes a canvas and the hair the painting medium (Fig. 1.37).

2

Colour

It is extremely important that hairdressers should understand the fundamental principles of colour theory because this is the necessary background that will enable them to use colour confidently in the salon. It is easy enough to colour a client's hair using client record cards and carefully following mixing instructions supplied with colouring products, but that is purely technical work and does not allow for creative skill. In order to exhibit creative flair and find the perfect colour to suit the client, the hairdresser must first have a comprehensive knowledge and understanding of colour itself. Not only will this knowledge instil confidence in the client, but also it will make life much easier for the hairdresser. If you know what you are talking about you will be confident in helping your clients make their colour decisions and you will have assurance about the results.

Colour choices are involved in many of the tasks the hairdresser undertakes including: choosing a warm or a cool colour appropriate to a client's skin tone; mixing colour tints; applying colours to the hair; neutralising colours; advising clients on colour choice; and even choosing salon lighting and using colour to decorate the salon.

2.1 COLOUR THEORY

In order to understand the nature of colour, it is important first to distinguish between the two different ways of producing colours – by addition and by subtraction.

Colour addition involves mixing together coloured lights. A good way to see this is by projecting different coloured spotlights to overlap on a white screen. If a red light is projected onto a green light, for instance, the colour produced is yellow (Fig. 2.1).

White light is a mixture of red, orange, yellow, green, blue and violet as

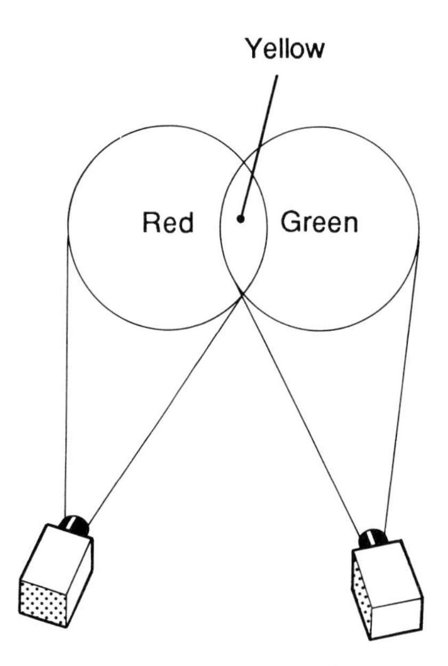

Fig. 2.1 Colour addition.

you may remember from your school days, when you were shown that a ray of sunlight, as it passes through a glass prism, separates out into these six colours of the rainbow. Adding red, orange, yellow, green, blue and violet lights therefore produces white light. You will become more aware of the effects of colour addition when you come to decorate your salon using coloured spotlights (see later in this chapter) or if you move into theatrical work.

Colour subtraction, using dyes or pigments, will be what you are dealing with more directly in your work when tinting hair in the salon or mixing colours in make-up.

The chemical nature of dyes and pigments is such that they selectively absorb light of some colours and reflect light of others. This is the process of colour subtraction, and it is in this way that all the colours seen in nature are produced. A red flower with green leaves (Fig. 2.2), for instance, does not generate light itself; it can only reflect light that comes from the sun or some other source of illumination, but the green pigment in the green leaves absorbs (i.e. subtracts) all the colours from this white light except green (which it reflects so the leaves appear green). The red pigment in the petals will absorb (i.e. subtract) all the colours except red, which it will reflect so that the petals appear red. Similarly, the different coloured objects you can see in the salon (the upholstery, the clients' clothes, etc.) are coloured differently because the pigments they contain absorb (i.e. subtract) different colours from the white light that is used to illuminate the salon and reflect the rest.

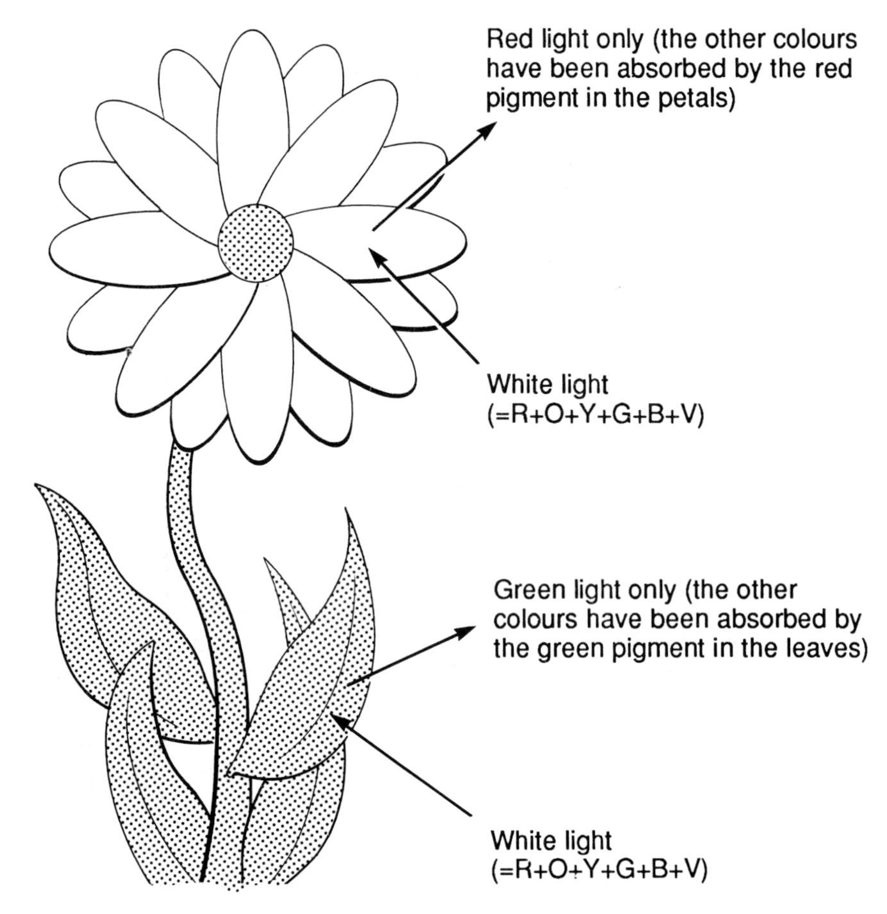

Fig. 2.2 Colour subtraction.

It follows that if we mix two different coloured pigments we produce a third colour which must absorb more of the colours in white light than either of the two original colours. Hence the visual result will be darker, ultimately black. This is why when you apply colour pigment to natural hair colour it will always result in a darker tone. You are mixing two colours together and working towards black. If you want to lighten the hair colour you need to mix the tint with a lightener (peroxide) before applying it.

Primary and secondary colours

Colour pigments are defined as either *primary* or *secondary* colours. We need to understand what these terms mean in order to master the principles of creating colours from mixtures of pigments.

The primary colours are *red*, *yellow* and *blue*. They are *pure* pigments, meaning that you cannot make up these colours from mixing others in the

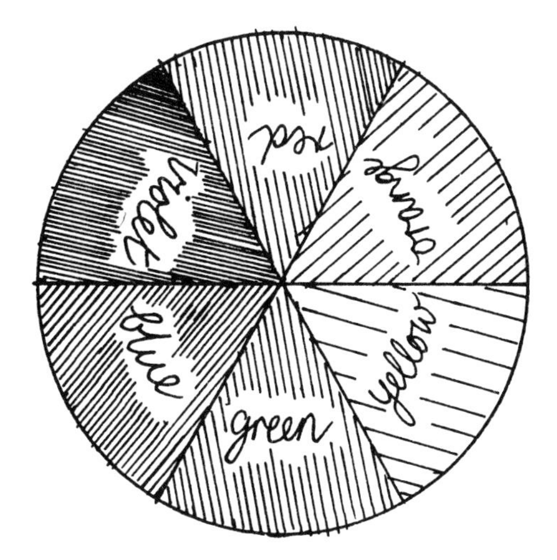

Fig. 2.3 Basic colour wheel.

palette, but that from these three colours, theoretically, all other colours can be mixed (depending on the proportions you use). An equal mixture of all three colours should produce black (but in practice a neutral grey usually results due to impure pigments).

Secondary colours are *orange*, *green* and *violet*. They are the result of two of the primary colours being mixed together to produce a third colour:

RED + YELLOW = ORANGE
YELLOW + BLUE = GREEN
BLUE + RED = VIOLET

These six hues form the basis of our colour wheel:

RED orange YELLOW green BLUE violet

2.2 THE COLOUR WHEEL

The colour wheel (Fig. 2.3) clearly gives the sequence of colours, and is a useful tool to use when determining which colours are complementary and which colours should be used to neutralise others. Keep the wheel beside you as you read the next section.

2.3 COMPLEMENTARY AND NEUTRALISING COLOURS

Complementary colours

Complementary colours, as painters call them, can be any two colours that sit opposite each other in the colour wheel. The term 'complementary' is used

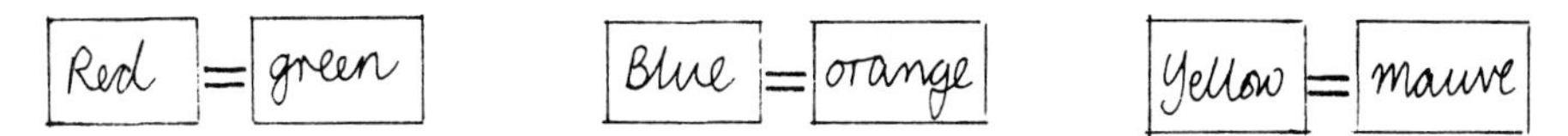

Fig. 2.4 Complementary colours.

because these two colours present a pleasing combination to the eye. If you look at a green square for any length of time and then glance away your eye seeks its complementary colour and you will see a red square as an after-image. Your eye is seeking to create a balance. We can see that the three primary colours are present in our two complementary colours:

e.g. RED + GREEN = RED + (YELLOW + BLUE).

Hence a mixture of red and green is a mixture of all three primary colours, and as we have already mentioned, the three primary colours mix to create a neutral grey. It is this neutralising that the eye is seeking when it throws up a red after-image to the green square. This rule of neutralising will apply for any pair of complementary colours. Figure 2.4 shows all the complementary colours.

Neutralising colours

The rules governing complementary colours apply equally in hairdressing only they are known as neutralising colours. This is because a treatment often leaves an unwanted colour on the hair that has to be neutralised by adding another. The colour to be added will always be the one opposite the unwanted colour on the colour wheel, and the hairdresser must find a product that contains that colour even though it will often have a quite different name.

For instance, if a client whose hair colour is dark brown has had highlights, the bleach will have stripped most of the black, brown and some of the red pigments from the hair leaving an unsatisfactory orangey/yellow shade. In order to neutralise this shade, the hairdresser finds the colour opposite it on the colour wheel, which is blue/violet. The hairdressing product which contains blue/violet is an 'ash' shade, so an ash toner applied to the hair will neutralise the colour giving the white/grey colour the client required.

It is important that the correct shade is used. In the above example, a toner with too much blue would create bright green highlights! That is why you must consult the colour wheel to find the exact shade directly opposite your unwanted colour.

Another example is if a client has requested a warm red tint on her mid-brown hair and the resulting colour has become too red. On the colour wheel we will see that a green should be applied, which from our hairdressing knowledge we know can be found in an 'ash brown' shade. This has a cooler greenish cast which will neutralise some of the red and result in a warm brown.

Identifying warm and cool colours

A common way of describing colours is to say whether they are warm or cool, and an easy way to determine whether a colour is warm or cool is to think of where it occurs in nature:

Warm colours are basically the colours you would associate with fire and the sun: yellow, red and oranges. Between the yellow and orange lies gold where our hairdressing gold browns and gold blondes slot in, and between orange and red we will find our warm auburn shades, coppers and chestnuts.

Cool colours, on the other hand, are colours you associate with the cold: blues, blue greens and violets. The violets and blues will give the ash tones to the hair and the greens will give the matt tones.

Warm and cool colours work as opposites just as neutralising colours do, so that on the colour wheel each warm colour has a cool colour as its opposite. For instance, a warm red is neutralised by a cool green, whereas a cool blue is neutralised by a warm yellow/gold colour (Fig. 2.5).

If a cool colour is mixed with a warm colour, then the proportion of the

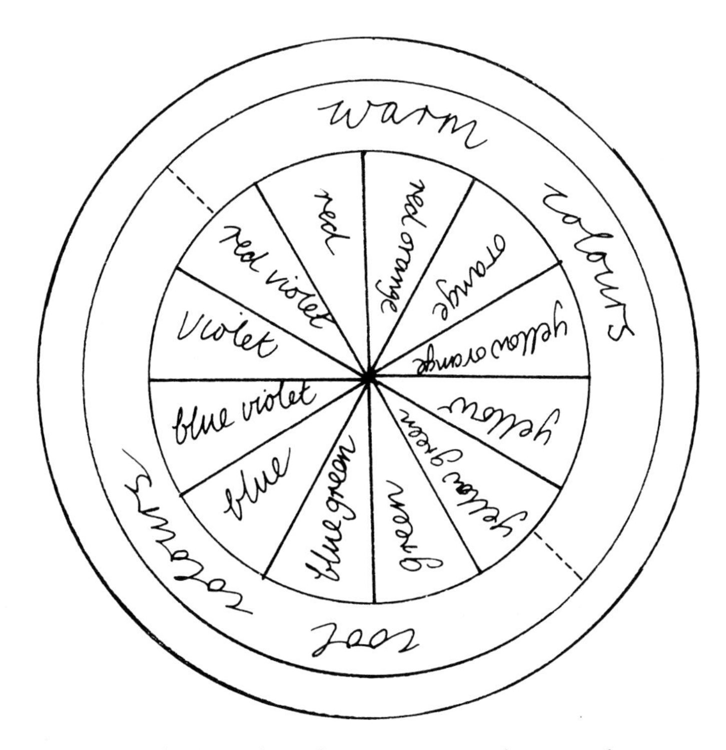

Fig. 2.5 Colour wheel used to determine neutralising and warm and cool colours.

pigment will determine the temperature of the shade, e.g. 75 per cent red with 25 per cent blue will give a warm mauve, but 75 per cent blue with 25 per cent red will give a cool violet.

Remember the effect of the hair!

When mixing pigments, the hairdresser must always remember, in addition to the general rules, that the colour of the hair itself can make a difference to the result. It is easy when the hair is stripped of colour and becomes white like a sheet of white paper; then a red dye of a particular intensity will come out just as it was mixed. However, the same dye on dark hair will give a very different result because the red combines with the hair colour. The base colour of the hair has to be taken into consideration as an additional colour that will play an important part in determining the resulting shade.

A good basic understanding of the colour wheel, mixing colours, warm and cool colours and neutralising colours coupled with a good basic knowledge of the hairdressing shade chart, will provide an excellent foundation for a competent, confident and creative stylist.

Shade charts

Different manufacturers offer shade charts with varying shades and names, but basically they are all the same. The base colours (or natural hair colourings) are numbered 1 to 10 from dark to light, 1 being black and 10 being the lightest blonde. These base colours are broken down into the four colour categories that are the pigments present in natural hair colouring: black, brown, red and yellow.

These base colours are usually listed down one side of the chart and across the top is a range of warm and cool shades that form an array of varying shades across the grid as they are mixed with the base colours.

It is interesting also to note the selling power of colour names. More often than not it is the name that sells the colour to the client rather than the colour itself. If the word summons up a desirable image it becomes extremely appealing; for instance, sunset has much more appeal to it than warm reddish brown.

2.4 COLOUR TERMS

Sometimes it can be confusing when different terms are used to explain what seems the same thing or when words that have a specific meaning in hairdressing are used in a more general way outside. Here are some common definitions used in hairdressing:

Shade – the basic overall colour of the hair.
Depth – the lightness or darkness of the colour.
Tone – the character of the colour – cool or warm.

Here are some common definitions used in art:

Harmonious colours are those that lie peacefully together, and that are on the same tonal plane; for instance, those that share any quarter of the colour wheel. Reds, oranges and yellowy oranges are harmonious.
Discordant colours are those that clash and are not on the same tonal plane, for instance, green and mauve.
Monochromatic – a single colour in all its tones from light to dark.
Tone – the quality of lightness or darkness present in a colour.

2.5 CHOOSING AND USING COLOUR

We cannot talk about colouring hair without also discussing the other important factors that should strongly influence the hairdresser's advice to the client: skin tones; eye colour; dress; and personality.

Colour tones

Nature is expert at matching skin tone to hair colourings, and even as we get older and the colour fades from our hair, so too does our skin tone change to complement it. The general rule is that tinted hair colour should only be a few shades different from the natural colour, but that is not to say that extremes cannot be successful. Peroxide blondes can be quite a striking fashion feature. The red, pink and green hair of the punk fashions also successfully produce a desirable image. But, on the other hand, dramatic colour change is only successful when the image is deliberate, and usually only on the young who have the personality, clothes and make-up to carry it off.

Extremes of colour change on the not-so-young can have grotesque results. The older client, for example, who insists on returning to the colour of her youth, which perhaps her memory has darkened a shade or two, leaves the salon looking ghoulish and stark. The middle-aged mum who is convinced that the golden locks of her teens will recapture the adventure in her life, only finds that somehow they do not quite look how she remembered, and really her now ruddy complexion looks quite hot and bothered against them. The hairdresser not only has to be a technical expert, but also a psychologist, and has to try to advise, guide and gently persuade clients. The hairdresser should have the knowledge to be able to identify the colouring of the client's skin tone, whether it is warm and has a golden undertone to the skin or cooler with a bluer undertone.

Warm tones usually consist of natural auburn, honey blonde, or reddish brown hair colourings and the skin can have freckles. Eye colourings are usually hazel-toned, or green speckled with yellow or brown.

Cool tones usually consist of natural ash blonde, dark brown or black hair colouring. The skin can have bluish or pinkish undertones to it, particularly in black or oriental skin tones. Eye colourings are usually cool blues, greeny-blues or dark browns.

Neutralising unwanted tones in the skin can be done in the same way as in hair, by choosing the appropriate colour from the opposite side of the colour wheel. For instance, a client who has a cool complexion bordering on a sallow appearance can look much more alive by having a warmer shade applied to the hair.

The opposite applies to a client who has a naturally red complexion. If cooler, ashen tones are applied to the hair it will help tone the red down, and give more of a balanced appearance.

Make-up can also lend a hand here as well. Although its general purpose should be to complement and enhance the skin tone, the choice of colour can also help to neutralise unwanted tones. For instance our client with the reddish complexion could help tone it down by choosing cooler eye shadows, e.g. greens/blues and a cooler lipstick which is bluish red rather than orangey red.

It takes time and experience to be able to assess what colours would or would not suit a client, except for the blatantly obvious combinations that you know would not look right, such as black skin tone with blonde hair or reddish skin tone with blonde hair or pure white skin tone with black hair. It is wise to begin by looking for the warm or cool tones in the client, as this is a good guide to help you make a suitable colour choice.

Personality and wardrobe

The client's personality and wardrobe should also be considered whenever possible in choosing hair colour. You might see the potential for bringing the quiet, introverted client out of herself, but you cannot make her into something she is not. Indeed she might be quite happy as she looks, so remember to communicate with her and do not get carried away.

The client's wardrobe is another important feature to bear in mind when choosing a colour. Most people have favourite colours they like to wear, and more or less intuitively they seem to choose the colours that suit their skin colourings. Use your knowledge of warm and cool colours and indeed harmonious and complementary colours to make your advice invaluable to them.

Here is an example of a client who wants a change and something to give her hair a lift. Her favourite wardrobe colours seem to be green, brown and dusky blues. Her base hair colour is six on the shade chart, with some coppery tones to it, and her skin colouring is warm. Her eyes are green/brown and speckled. All the features should indicate warmth, with the cooler dusky blues of the wardrobe complementing them, so your advice as to the lift she desires would best tend towards warm red lowlights or, depending on how much lift she was actually thinking of, perhaps a whole head tint. Always remember, though, if the client is not totally sold on the idea then suggest a semi-permanent first, so she can adjust to the colour change first.

Colour symbolism and expression

Colour is subjective. Personal favourites or dislikes depend upon individual responses and emotions, but in general different colour preferences do seem to suggest an overall pattern of responses that seems to have stayed the same over time. The ancient Egyptians' use of colour had strong symbolic meaning representing the gods, whereas the Tudors used colour to signify wealth and power in the clothes they wore. Today, colour is used more generally to convey messages; for instance, red indicates danger, and green indicates go. It also helps us to express emotions as in 'green with envy' or the 'lonesome blues'. More than this, it has the power to influence our emotions – it can make us feel uncomfortable, hot, cold or peaceful. This is important to remember when embarking on a colour scheme for general public use and is covered more in Chapter 5, Salon Design.

The colour of the clothes we wear can reflect our personality. Bold colours such as red and yellow suggest an extrovert, whereas black or brown might indicate more of an introvert who does not want to attract attention. Here are some examples of colours and what they traditionally signify:

Red. The colour of blood. A hot colour, it has the longest wavelength (infra-red) and is the fastest colour in catching the eye and the most emotional. It can be provocative and arousing when used.
Orange. This word did not exist in English until the first oranges were brought here in the 10th and 11th Centuries. A hot colour associated with flames, and the setting sun, it is also associated with energy.
Yellow. A cheerful colour and the colour of the sun. It has vibrancy and is associated with truth.
Green. The colour of both life and destruction (nature, rebirth of spring as well as mould, decay, vomit, envy). It is a peaceful colour to the eye and is often used to decorate hospitals, dental surgeries, etc.
Blue. A cool colour that is soothing. It can indicate sadness and depression, but also faith and contentment.
Violet/purple. It has the shortest wavelength (ultra-violet). It can be a sensual colour and can indicate depth of feeling, mystery and can represent death.

Seasonal colours

In Itten's *The Art of Colour*, the four seasonal palettes are perfectly illustrated. Pale spring colours, predominantly yellows, pinks, blues and lilacs, represent anticipation of the vibrancy of summer. Summer colours are warm, pure and strong and have the intensity that represents full bloom: oranges, reds, leaf-greens, warm mauves. Autumn has the warmth of dying summer colours, tawny oranges, browns, autumn leaf. Winter's palette represents the stillness of the season: greys, blacks, icy blues and whites leave the right cool impression.

2.6 LIGHTING

The important point about lighting in the salon is to strike a balance between creating the right atmosphere so it is not too stark and bright, and allowing the clients the visibility to actually see what is being done to them!

The tinting area must have good illumination, to be able to see the correct colour choice. The best lighting for this is obviously natural daylight, but it is not always possible to get enough daylight in this particular area. Instead, either 'natural' fluorescent tubes or 'daylight' electric light bulbs will give a good simulation of natural daylight and reflect reasonably true colours. Ordinary electric light bulbs are usually tungsten bulbs and have a strong orange hue which will not only dramatically affect the appearance of the natural colour of the clients' hair before tinting, but also misguide your colour choice. The same applies to 'white' fluorescent light. This will reflect a cold, bluish hue across the hair and also affect the correct choice of colour.

Other areas of the salon should have softer lights. Many salons have concealed lighting around the walls, with extra illumination by the addition of spotlights. If coloured spotlights are used to give a particular effect, then a slightly different colour mix must be observed. As has already been mentioned in the section on Colour Theory, additive colour or the colours in the form of projected light, when all added together, make white light. When lights of the three primary colours (red, green and blue) are mixed together different results are produced from when colour pigments are mixed together. For instance, red and green lights projected together will result in a yellow light, and green and blue lights projected together will result in cyan (blue) light.

Obviously, the lights will affect the colour of everything within their range including hair, skin, clothes, objects, and surfaces. Care should be taken, because although to some degree light could be used to give a dramatic effect and could be a lively feature or gimmick in the salon, it should only be treated as such and carefully placed.

2.7 QUESTIONS ON COLOUR

Complete the following sentences:

(1) In colour pigments, the three primary colours are ....

(2) The colour made when the three primary colours are mixed together as pigments is ....

(3) In coloured lights the three primary colours are ....

(4) The colour made when all three primary colour lights are mixed together is ....

(5) The monochromatic scale describes the ....
.... of a colour.

(6) In colour pigment mixing a red and a blue will make the colour ......

(7) The secondary colours are those mixed from two of the primary colours and they are ....

(8) In the colour wheel yellow/green is complementary to ....

(9) Complementary colours in art terms are the same as ....
.... in hairdressing terms.

(10) Too much orangey yellow in the hair can be neutralised by applying a .... colour which you can find in a .... toner.

(11) Colours associated with warmth are ....
.... and with cold are ....

(12) The colour made by a green and a red light projected together is .....

3

Features Influencing Hair Design

The shape of the face is the most important feature to consider when choosing a suitable style. However, there are other factors that can also influence styling decisions, and it is best to study a client's facial and body features before making any final decisions.

3.1 FACE SHAPES

Face shape is one of the most important features influencing any decisions about choosing a suitable hair style. It can be a difficult task to identify accurately the shape of a person's face because not everyone has a 'pure' face shape and each face is individual. Also, many people have a combination of two shapes, so the most dominant shape has to be identified.

Some people are oblivious of the fact that faces actually differ in shape, but the more enlightened people, although they know that face shapes are different, still find it difficult to identify which shape is which. It is a skill that has to be practised. A good starting-point is to be able to identify your own face shape, and there are different exercises that make it easier. One way is to pull back all your hair from your face and hold a mirror in front of you with one hand, then using a piece of chalk or felt-tip pen to draw round your mirrored face shape on the mirror. This will give a good indication of the basic shape (Fig. 3.1).

Another exercise that can be done with a partner is to cut out a small square (2 cm × 2 cm) from the centre of a small piece of card and then ask your partner to hold all the hair back off her face. Then look through the small square with one eye at your partner's face so that the square just encases her face shape, from the hair line to in front of the ears and the jaw line. Once the shape is framed within the square it is much easier to identify the actual overall shape. Once this skill has been mastered, it is then just a question of practice to be able to identify a person's face shape (Fig. 3.2).

Many people do have face shapes which are a combination, but once you

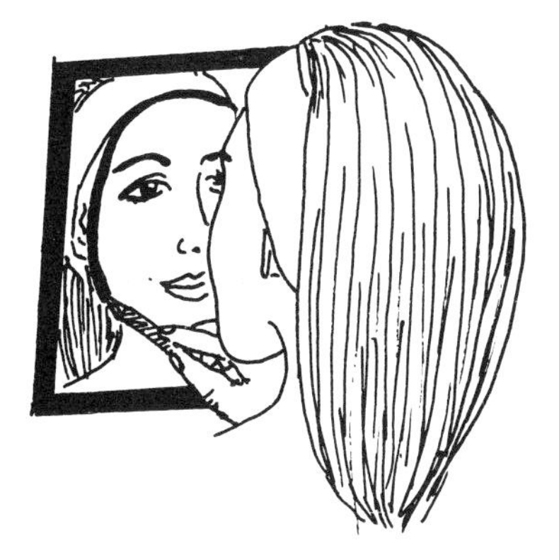

Fig. 3.1 Drawing your own face shape on a mirror.

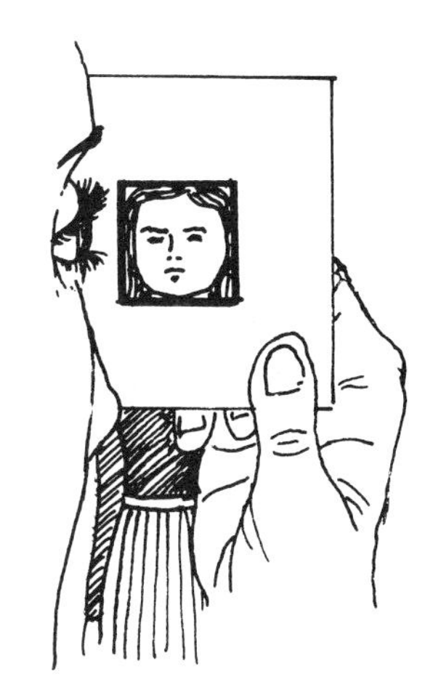

Fig. 3.2 Framing the face to determine its shape.

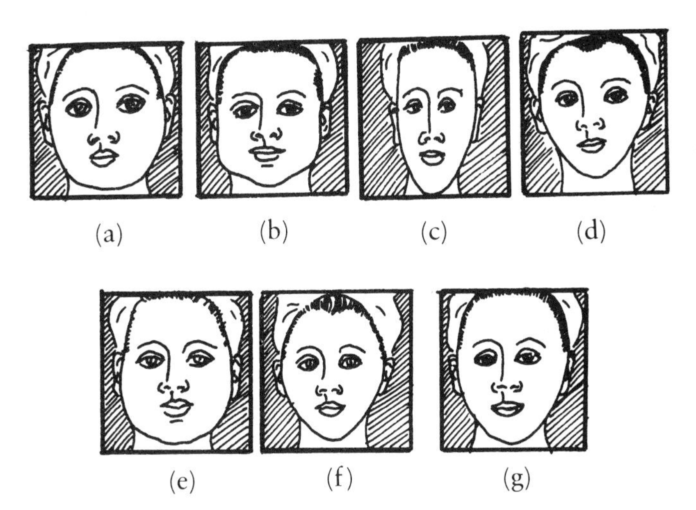

Fig. 3.3 The seven basic face shapes: (a) round; (b) square; (c) long; (d) heart; (e) pear; (f) diamond; (g) oval.

can identify the basic face shapes then it is just a case of identifying which is dominant. This is the one that needs to be considered when choosing a suitable hair style. It is also worth remembering that as a person ages the face shape changes. As a person enters into the middle years (40–50) the jaw line usually becomes heavier taking on more of a 'jowled' appearance, so that what might have been an appropriate hair style earlier on in life does not necessarily follow through to later in life. It is also important to make sure that whatever the final decision is, the style is one that the person feels comfortable with and is manageable, as well as suiting the face shape.

There are seven basic shapes of faces. These are shown in Fig. 3.3.

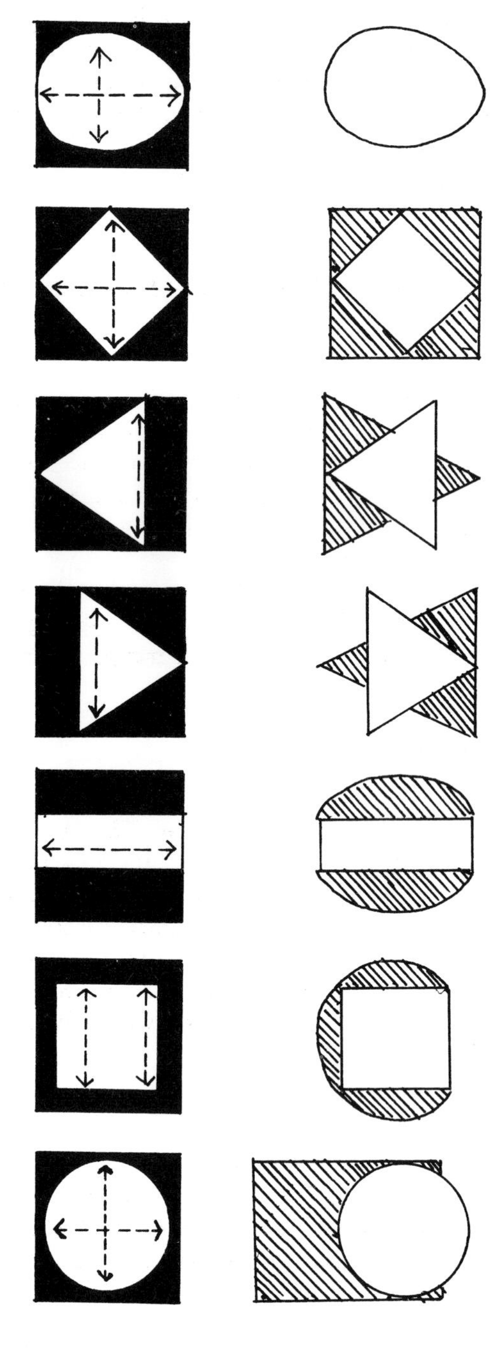

Fig. 3.4 Simplified face shapes. The shaded areas counterbalance the face shapes and illustrate the shape of the hair style needed to balance the face.

The oval face shape is considered to be the most in proportion and evenly balanced, therefore when we design hair styles we are usually trying to create an evenly balanced feature similar to the oval shape. If the face shape is out of proportion then we have to balance it with a hair style that counter-balances the odd shape to produce an oval appearance. To illustrate this look at Fig. 3.4. The shapes are simplified into basic forms, and the counter-balancing shapes are shaded in to make them oval. We can see from this the shapes of the hair styles that we need to use in order to gain proportion and balance, and complement the face shape.

Suitable and unsuitable styles for each face shape

Round face shape (Fig. 3.5)

The contour of the face is usually quite circular and the proportions are too equal, the width being practically the same as the length. The aim of complementing this face shape and counterbalancing the roundness is to choose a style that will square off the face and give a slimmer appearance. The best styles to do this are those that give height but no width; those with partings; and angular and asymmetrical styles.

Styles that are best *avoided* as they emphasise the roundness of the face shape are those that have a round shape themselves – soft, curly styles or short, cropped styles, or those that add width. Full fringes only emphasise the roundness of the jaw line.

Square face shape (Fig. 3.6)

The contour of this face is very angular, and the width, particularly at the cheekbones or jaw line, is the distorted proportion. The aim of choosing a suitable style is to soften the squareness and make the appearance rounder. Hair coming softly onto the face, rounded at the temples and cheekbones, soft cascading curls framing the face and soft asymmetrical styles also help to break up the squareness. Styles that should be *avoided* are any angular or geometric cuts, or styles finishing sharply at the jaw line. Short cropped or spiky styles or hair drawn away from the face will only emphasise the squareness.

Long face shape (Fig. 3.7)

The long face shape is generally thin in appearance and the most obvious proportion of the face is the length. The aim is to balance the shape out by adding width to the sides, but without adding any height. Styles that are best suited are layered cuts that are scrunch-dried adding fullness at the sides, or soft perms. Fringes can also help to widen the face, and soft asymmetrical styles help to fill it out.

Styles that are best *avoided* are those that are long and straight, short cropped styles, and styles that give height and no width.

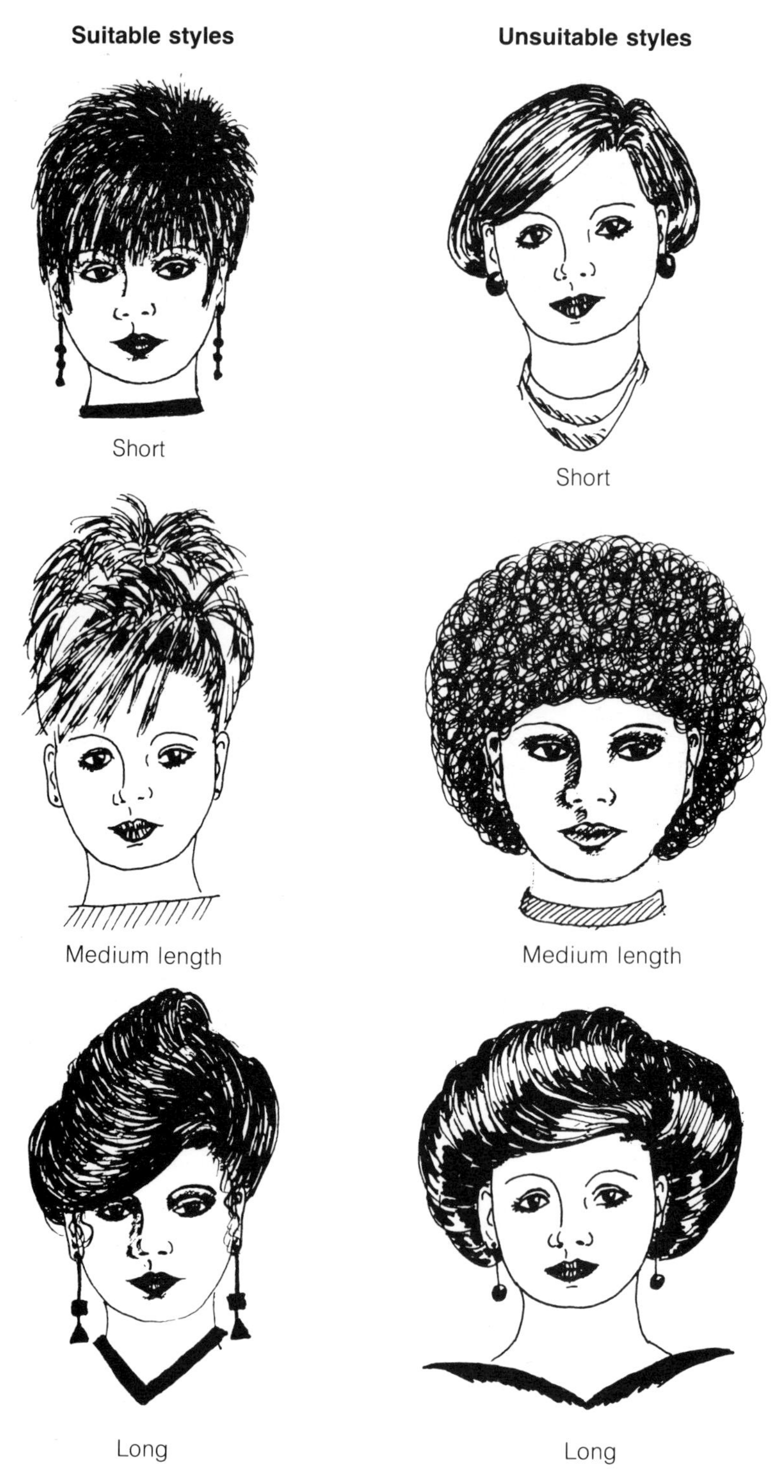

Fig. 3.5 Suitable and unsuitable styles for a round face shape.

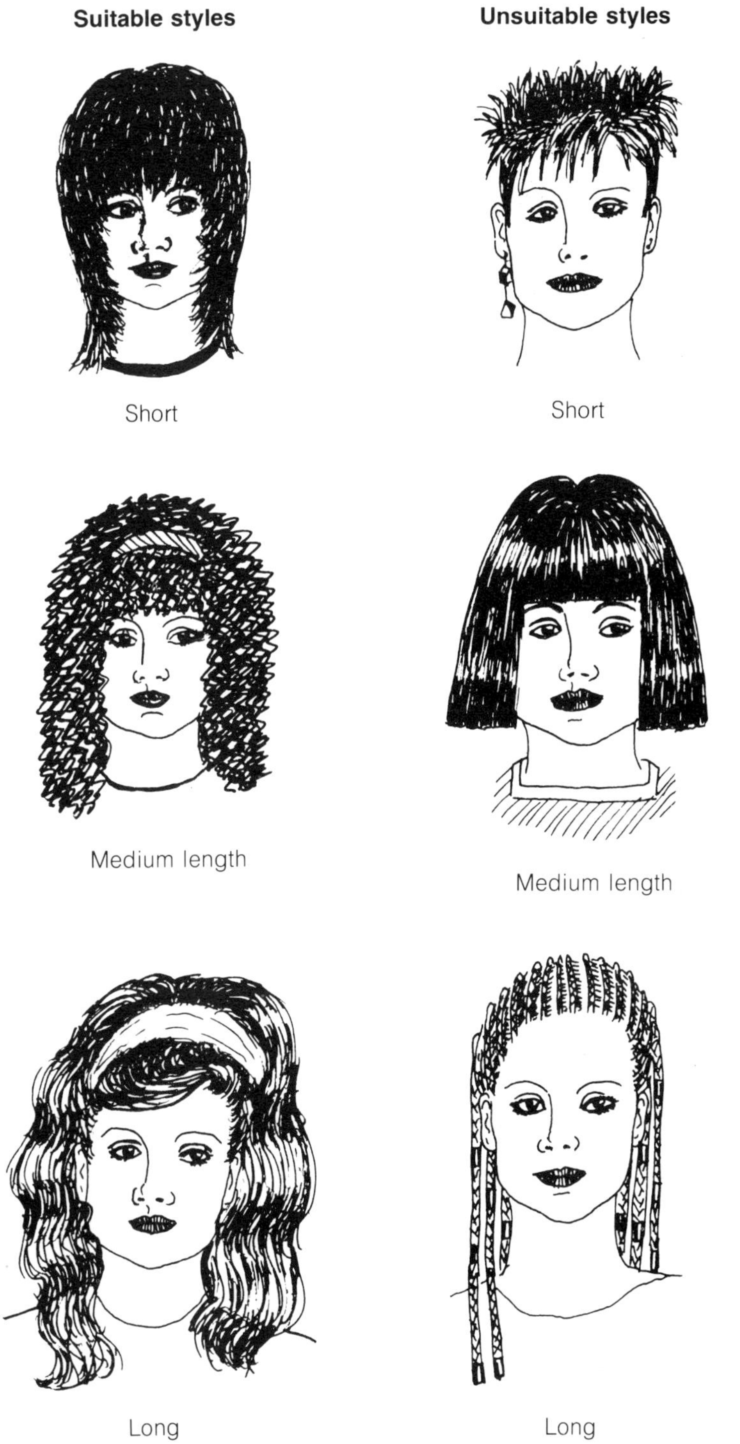

Suitable styles | **Unsuitable styles**

Short

Short

Medium length

Medium length

Long

Long

Fig. 3.6 Suitable and unsuitable styles for a square face shape.

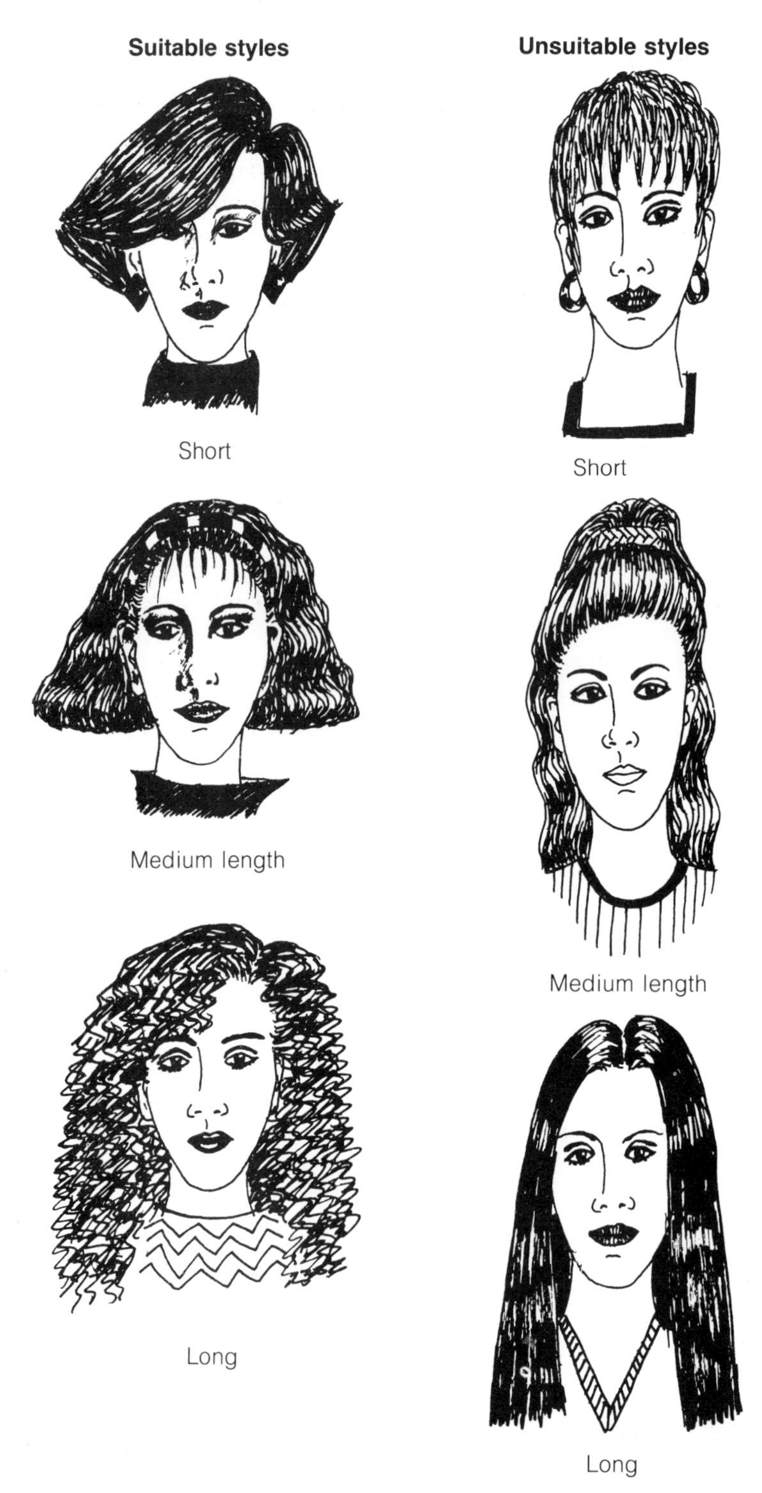

Fig. 3.7 Suitable and unsuitable styles for a long face shape.

Heart face shape (inverted triangle) (Fig. 3.8)

The contour of the heart face shape is not too far removed from the desired oval shape except that the width between the cheekbones is too great for the length of the face and the shape of the chin is sharper and usually too pointed. The styles which counterbalance this shape are pear-shaped styles – those that are narrow at the sides and give width at the jaw line. These styles draw attention to the jaw line and help widen the chin.

Styles to *avoid* are, obviously, styles that give width at the cheekbones, or short cropped styles, or styles that are off the face and give height.

Pear face shape (triangular) (Fig. 3.9)

The pear face shape has a heavy jaw line. The proportions are unbalanced with the width at the temples being far less than the width at the jaw line. This results in a 'jowled' appearance. The aim in choosing suitable hair styles is to counterbalance the shape with heart shape or inverted triangular hair shapes. Styles that add width at the cheekbones and temples, but without adding too much height and those that are soft around the nape area are suitable.

Styles to *avoid* are, obviously, those that add width at the jaw line, such as bobs, or styles that are too short or spiky. Also, if the hair is taken away from the front hairline it will draw attention to the lack of proportion in the width between the forehead and the jaw.

Diamond face shape (Fig. 3.10)

The contour of the diamond face shape is very similar to that of the heart shape face, except that the forehead narrows more and the overall appearance is too angular and sharp. The proportions are quite balanced, but the temples and jaw line need to be filled out more and softened. Styles that best counterbalance this shape are rounded and add width at the temples and jaw line, but are narrow or short at the sides.

Styles to *avoid* are those that emphasise the angular shape, such as geometric cuts, or styles that add height or width. Shorter layered cuts will also emphasise the angular shape of the face.

Oval face shape (Fig. 3.11)

The contour of an oval face shape is well balanced and even, and is similar to the perfect proportions of an egg shape. It is therefore the most desired face shape, and most hair styles suit it, although the aim when choosing should be to maintain the oval appearance.

3.2 FACIAL CHARACTERISTICS

It seems that most of the time when a style consulting session is going on between hairdresser and client, the decisions that are made are only made

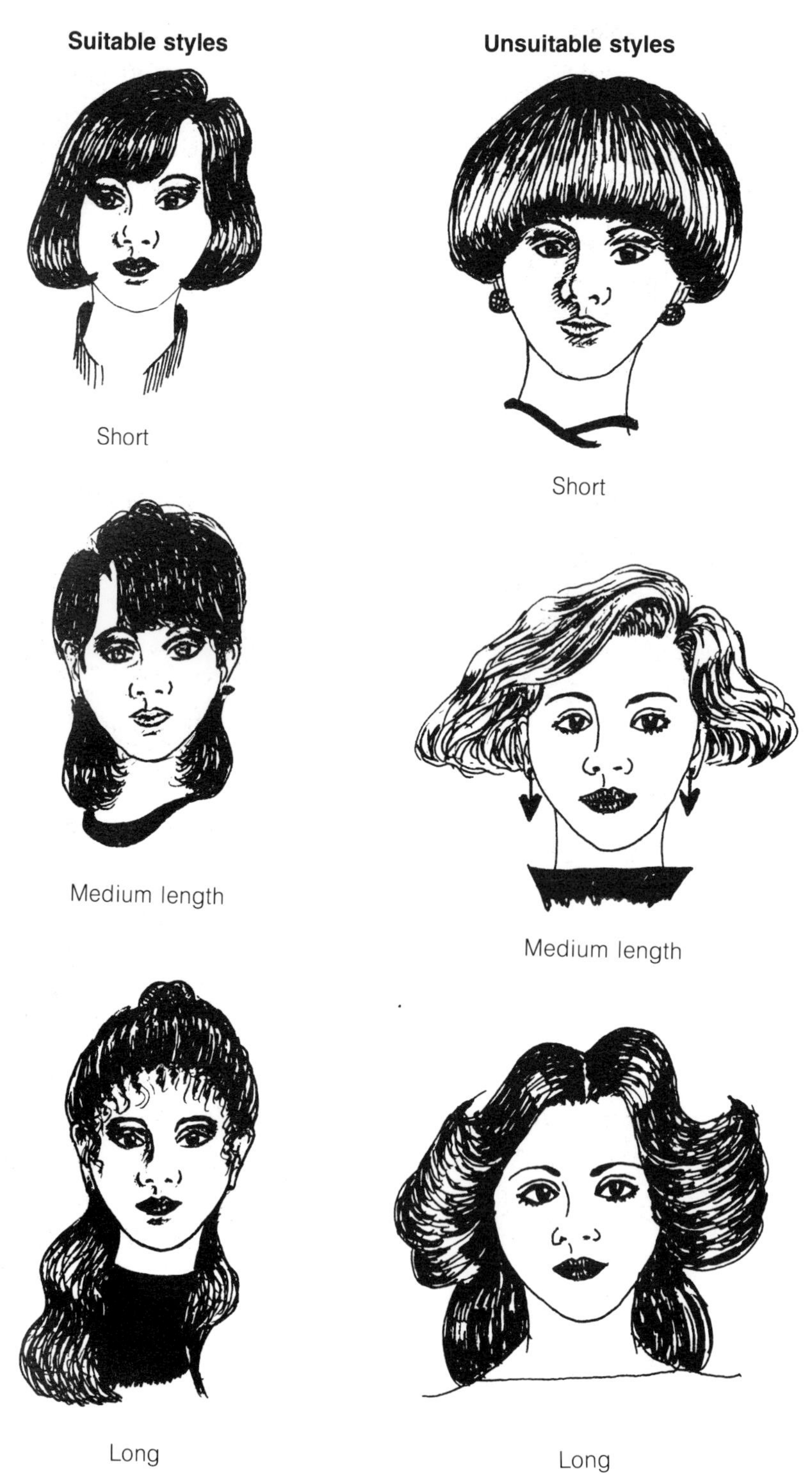

Fig. 3.8 Suitable and unsuitable styles for a heart face shape.

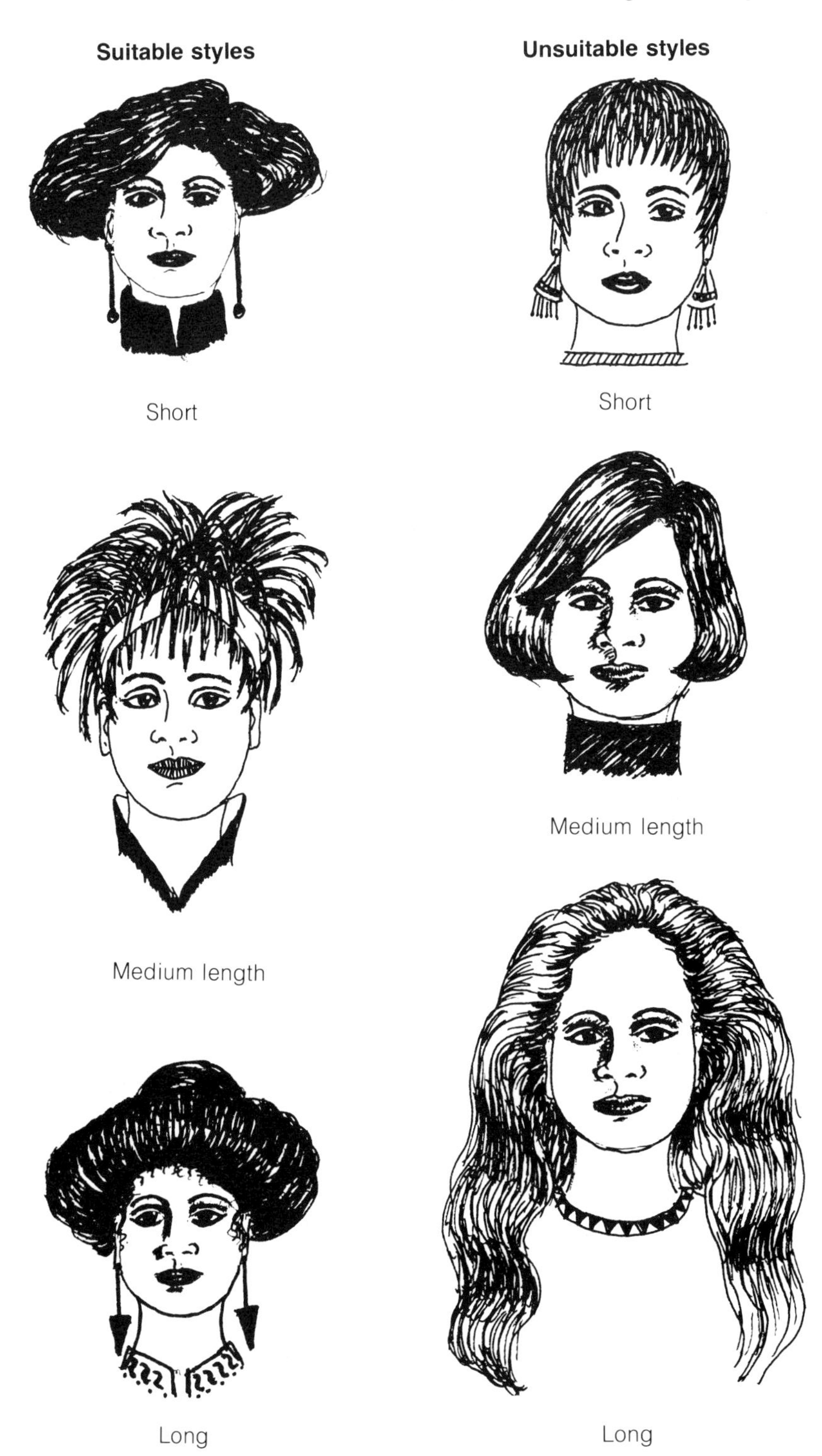

Fig. 3.9 Suitable and unsuitable styles for a pear face shape.

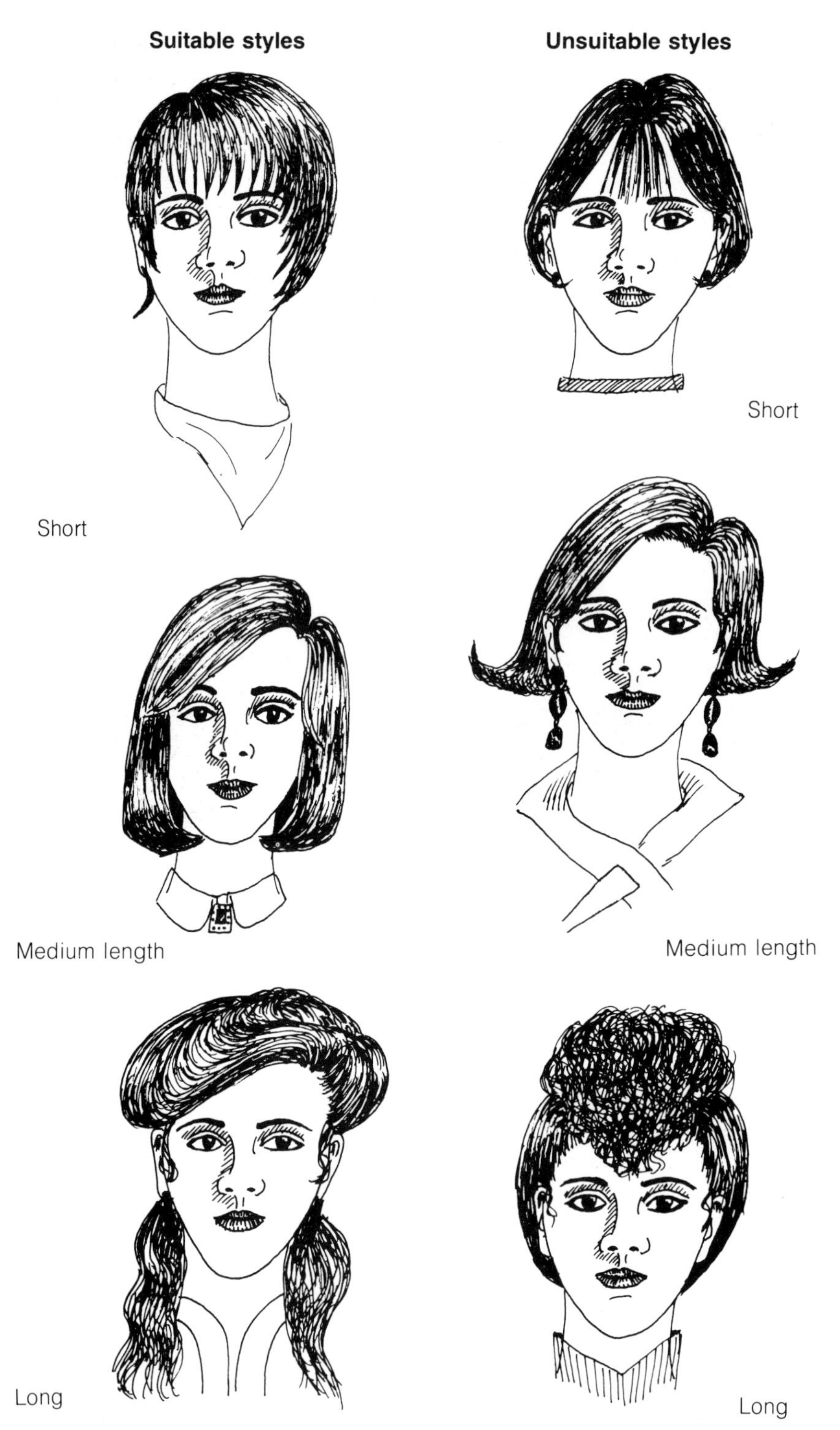

Fig. 3.10 Suitable and unsuitable styles for a diamond face shape.

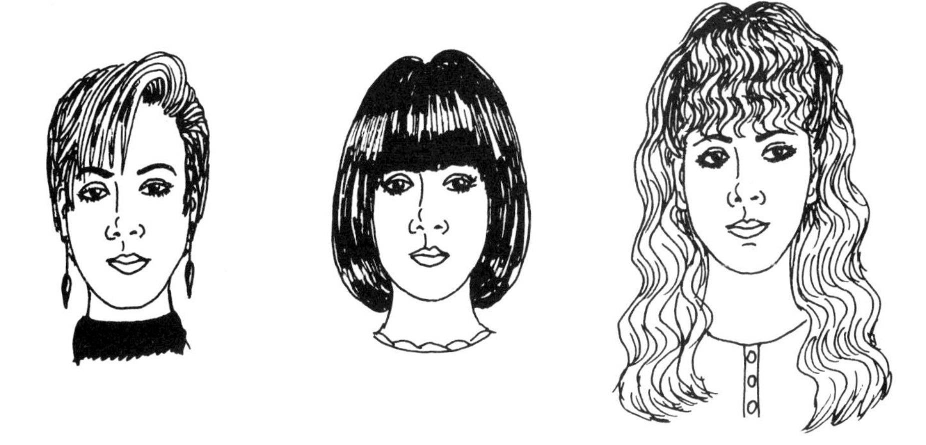

Fig. 3.11 Suitable styles for an oval face shape (short, medium length, and long hair).

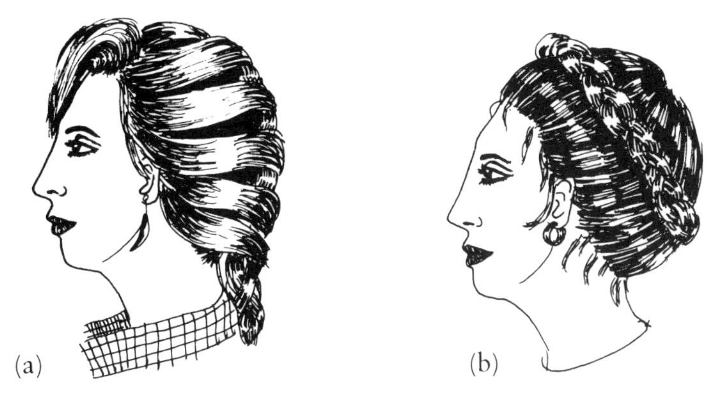

Fig. 3.12 (a) Suitable and (b) unsuitable styles for a convex profile.

from one view, the front, but it is important to remember that the head is a three-dimensional object and like any other object it has sides and a back that also have to be considered.

Profiles

Convex profile (Fig. 3.12)

The characteristic features of a convex profile are usually a small slanting forehead and small slanting chin that almost blends into the neck without any definite shape. Both of these features draw attention to the nose, emphasising its shape and making its size look out of proportion. In order to

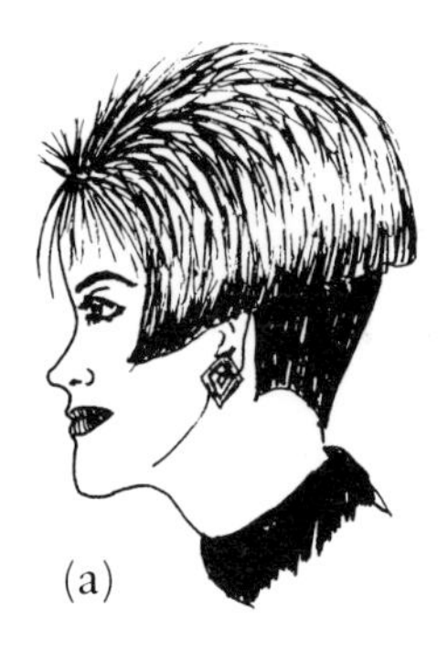

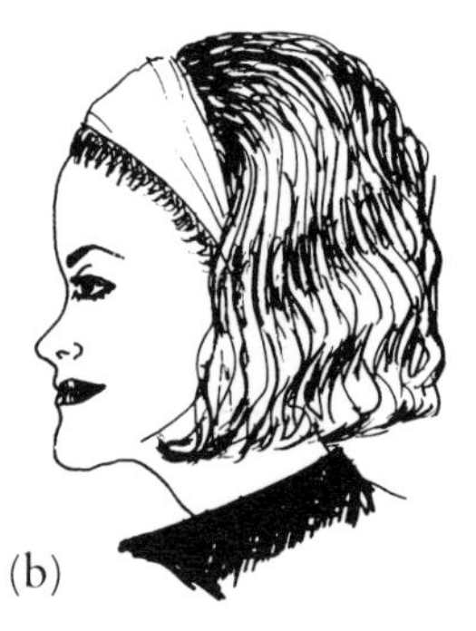

Fig. 3.13 (a) Suitable and (b) unsuitable styles for a concave profile.

counterbalance this profile, as best as possible, the convex line needs to be broken down. Hair styles that are best suited to this task are those that have curlier, fuller fringes, styles that have fullness at the front but are flat at the crown, or that come softly onto the face.

Styles that are best *avoided* are those that accentuate the convex line or draw diagonals with the nose, such as styles where the hair is drawn off the face into a top-knot, or styles that draw attention to the jaw line, or any style where the hair needs to be taken off the face.

Concave profile (Fig. 3.13)

The characteristic features of the concave profile are a large, rounded forehead and a protruding chin which detracts from the size of the nose, so that the whole profile gives the appearance of caving in. In order to camouflage this profile, as best as possible, the emphasis needs to be placed on making the nose look more in proportion. Styles are best that add height on the crown, and softly fall onto the forehead, or that add fullness at the sides and finish below the ear level.

Styles that are best *avoided* as they would emphasise the forehead and chin are those that require the hair to be taken off the forehead, or that finish at chin level.

Head shapes (Fig. 3.14)

Just as everybody has an individual face shape, so too is the head shape individual. This is an important feature to consider particularly when the client is deciding on a short hair style. The curve of the bones of the skull will affect the shape of the cut and whether it will complement the shape of the whole head. Sometimes it is difficult to see the true shape of the head, but feeling it with your hands should give a clear indication of the shape.

There are also other details to take notice of. Sebaceous cysts or warts can

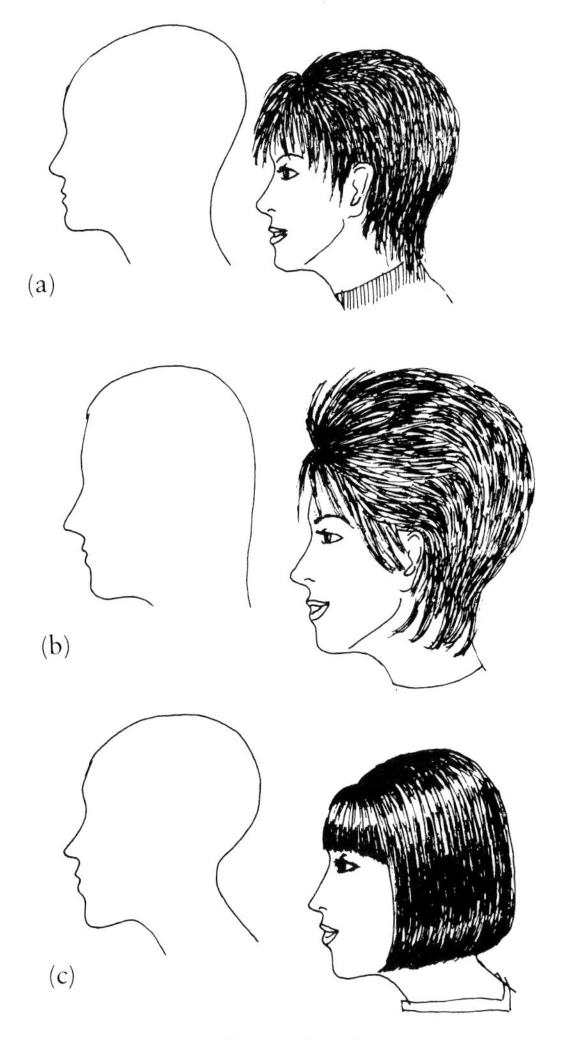

Fig. 3.14 Suitable styles for different head shapes: (a) in proportion; (b) flattened; (c) too curved.

look unsightly if the hair is cut too short so that they protrude through, and scar tissues can also stand out.

Foreheads

The forehead can affect the choice of a hair style to some extent, particularly if its size is too out of proportion with the rest of the face, i.e. too small or narrow, or too big. Proportionally, the distance between the hairline and the eyes should be nearly the same as the distance between the eyes and the end of the nose.

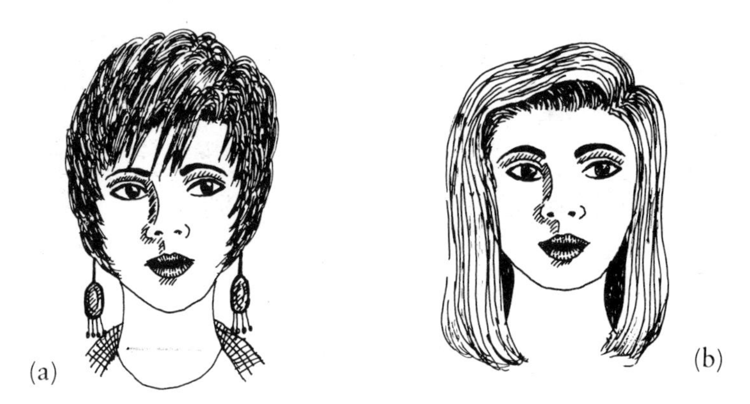

Fig. 3.15 (a) Suitable and (b) unsuitable styles for a narrow forehead.

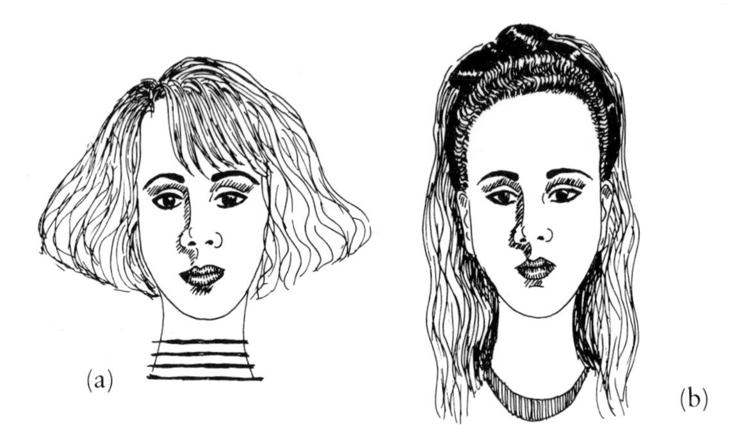

Fig. 3.16 (a) Suitable and (b) unsuitable styles for a large forehead.

Narrow forehead (Fig. 3.15)

In order to camouflage a narrow forehead it is best to aim for styles that add height, and are narrow at the sides, with a wispy fringe falling softly onto the forehead.

Styles to *avoid* are those that require a heavy, full fringe or styles that are drawn off the face. These will only emphasise the narrowness of the forehead.

Large forehead (Fig. 3.16)

A large forehead can look quite out of proportion. The best method of minimising the size is to aim for hair styles with full or asymmetric fringes, and for styles that add width to the head but definitely no height.

Styles that are best *avoided* are those that demand the hair to be taken off the face and any styles that give height.

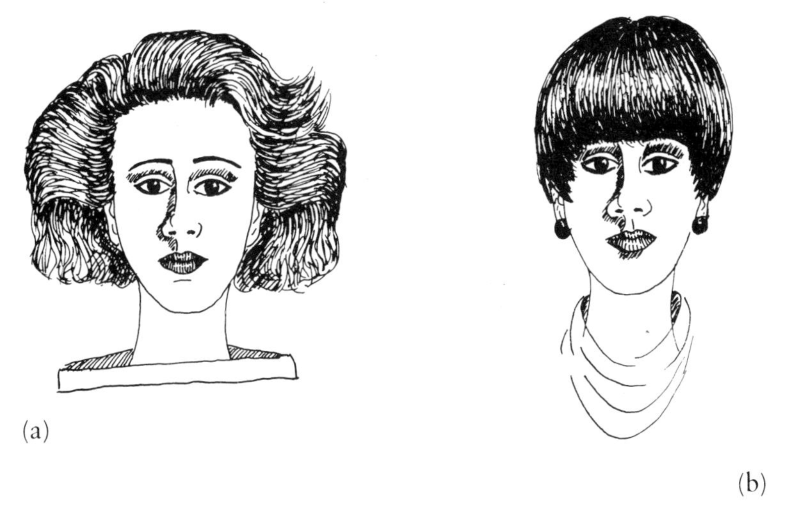

Fig. 3.17 (a) Suitable and (b) unsuitable styles for close-set eyes.

Eyes

To be in proportion, the space between the eyes should be of sufficient size so that an imaginary third eye could be easily placed there. If this is not so and they are either too close together or too wide apart, then carefully applied make-up can act as a counterbalance, and a suitable choice of hair style can also help. It is worth remembering that styles with full fringes act as a frame around the eyes and draw attention to them, so make sure that this is the desired effect when discussing such a style with the client.

Close-set eyes (Fig. 3.17)

The position of close-set eyes makes the nose look big, so carefully applied eye make-up extending outward helps. A hair style that added width and fullness at the top and sides, particularly extending the hair out from the sides, and also a light, asymmetrical fringe would help to draw the eyes apart more. It would also help to draw more attention to the jaw line.

Styles to *avoid* are those that are narrow at the sides, or cropped short, or styles that come onto the face, especially around the temple area.

Eyes set wide apart (Fig. 3.18)

The position of the eyes when they are wide apart gives a similar appearance to that of a heart-shaped face, with too much width at the sides. Eye make-up applied to the nose side of the eyelid will help diminish the width. The appropriate hair style would be narrow at the sides, without too much height and full at the jaw line, drawing attention away from the eyes. Also a soft line coming onto the face would be suitable.

Styles to *avoid* are those that extend away from the top or sides, or perms

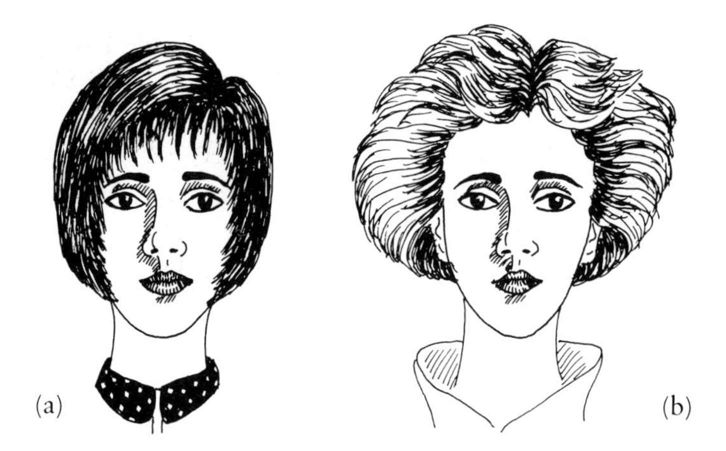

Fig. 3.18 (a) Suitable and (b) unsuitable styles for eyes set wide apart.

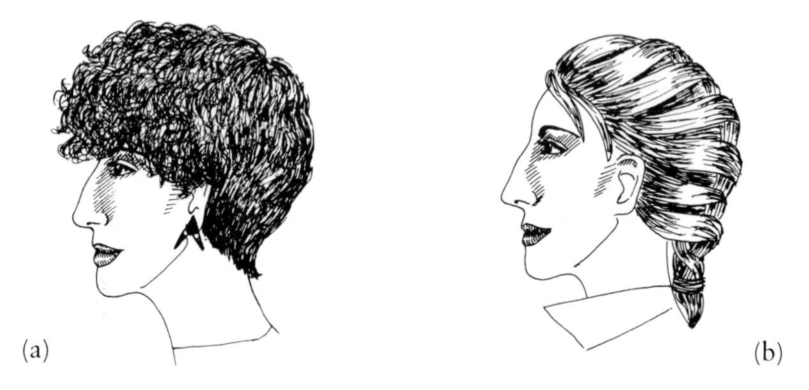

Fig. 3.19 (a) Suitable and (b) unsuitable styles for large noses.

that give fullness, short crops or a style where the hair is drawn away from the face.

Noses (Fig. 3.19)

A large nose can mean absolute misery and a life-time of painful self-consciousness to some people. Although plastic surgery is becoming more accessible and tricks of make-up can help diminish the size by drawing attention to the eyes and lips, a suitable choice of hair style can also contribute in the art of camouflaging. It is best to choose a hair style that will balance the whole head, adding fullness at the front and forehead, with no height at the crown as this would draw an imaginary diagonal line through to the nose. A style that gave either fullness at the jaw line or followed the shape of the head and neck would also be suitable.

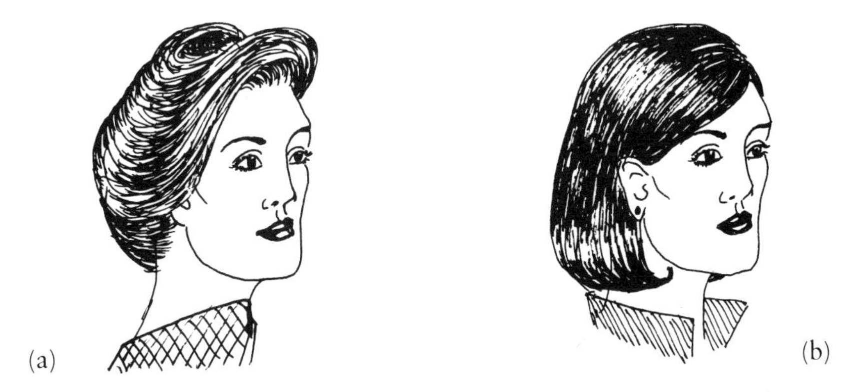

Fig. 3.20 (a) Suitable and (b) unsuitable styles for large jaws.

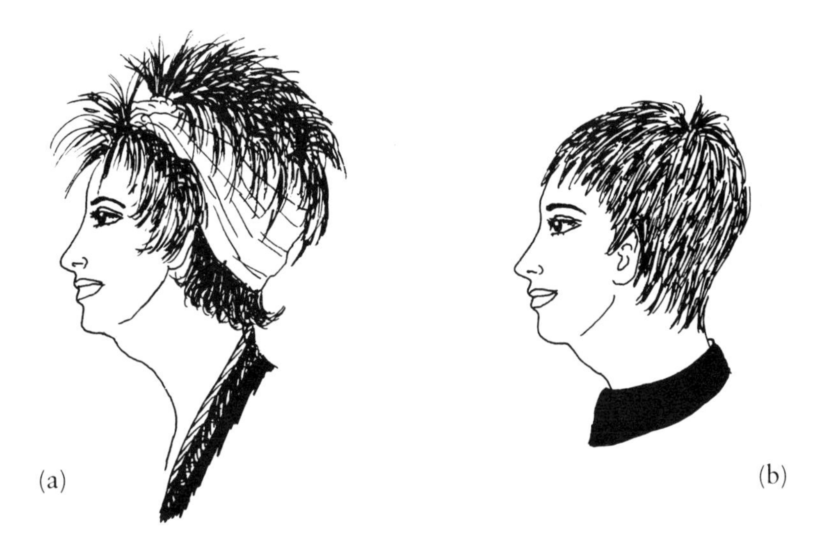

Fig. 3.21 (a) Suitable and (b) unsuitable styles for flabby chins.

Styles to *avoid* are short cropped styles, those with centre partings as these would act as indication lines to the nose, or styles that add too much height at the crown.

Jaws and chins (Figs 3.20 and 3.21)

Large jaws and chins both need similar styles to help camouflage them as best as possible, although they are both strong definite lines in the contour of the face and neck. Styles that best help a person with a large, protruding jaw are those that add width to the sides and back so as to balance the head. Suitable styles distract from the jaw line and bring more attention to the other

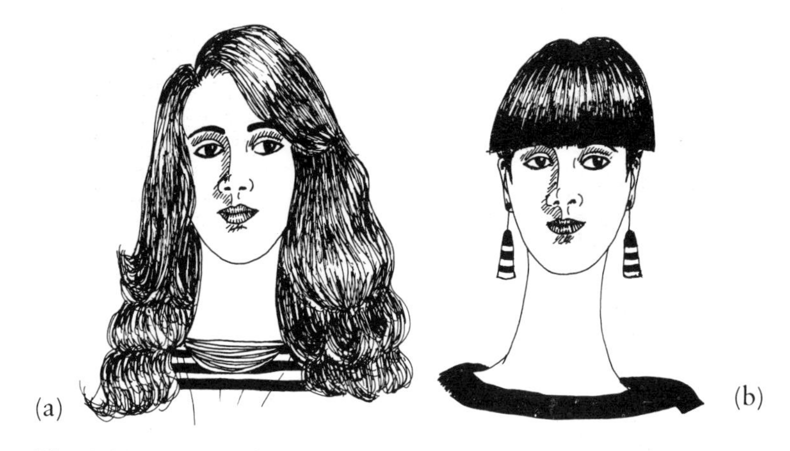

Fig. 3.22 (a) Suitable and (b) unsuitable styles for long necks.

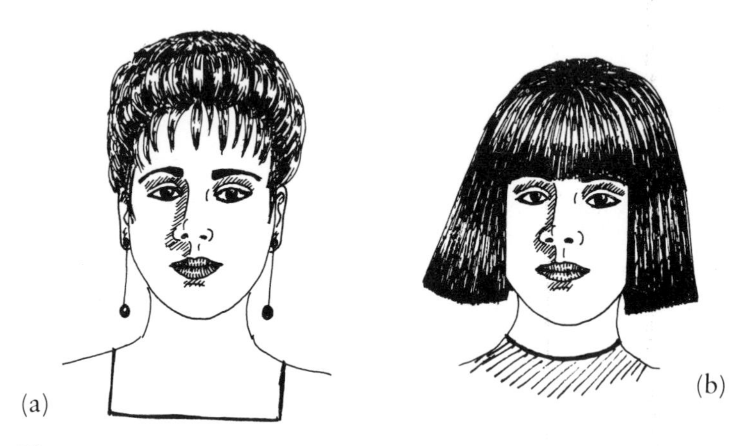

Fig. 3.23 (a) Suitable and (b) unsuitable styles for short necks.

features, such as the eyes and forehead. A flabby chin line can also be camouflaged to some extent by wearing styles that add fullness on the top but are narrow at the sides.

Styles that are best *avoided* for both features are those that emphasise the jaw line or contour of the head, such as hair cut close to the head, or hair drawn up in a plait or top-knot.

Necks (Figs 3.22 and 3.23)

We are led to believe that it is a desirable feature to have a neck that is reasonably long, probably because it has been associated with being graceful and it certainly does help in setting off the shape of the head. The length of

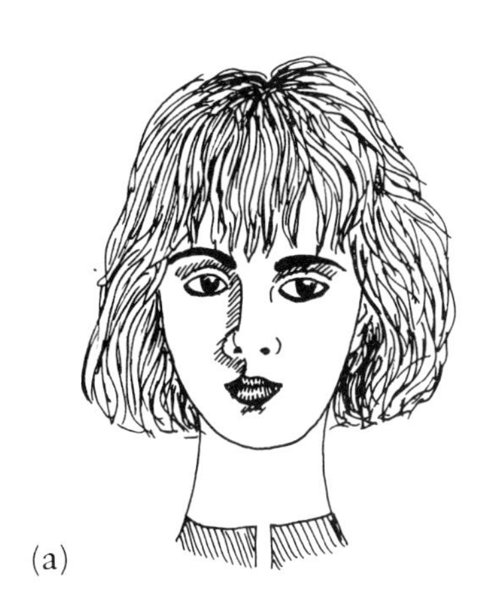

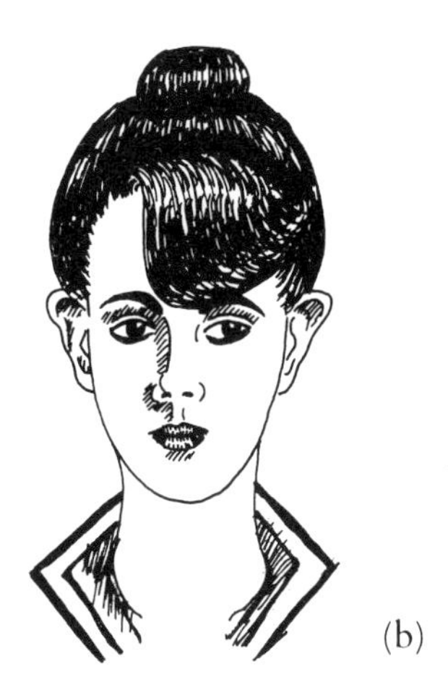

Fig. 3.24 (a) Suitable and (b) unsuitable styles for protruding ears.

the neck can also affect the overall look of a hair style, particularly if the neck is extremely long or too short. The wrong choice of style can make the head and neck look completely out of proportion with the rest of the body. A long 'swan' neck can look elegant if the hair is in a fuller, longer style without any added height, but it looks too long if worn with a particularly short hair style, or if the hair is swept up off the neck.

A short neck can be made to appear longer if the hair style has fullness and height on top of the head. It should be narrow at the sides and into the nape. If the client has long hair and does not want to wear it short, then the same effect can be gained by wearing it swept off the neck into a style on top of the head. But a short neck can look like a 'bull' neck if the hair is left to hang long or is in a style that finishes at the jaw line.

Ears (Fig. 3.24)

Protruding ears can be a menace with some hair styles. For instance they can stick out of straight, sleek styles, or look even bigger with short styles. The only way of camouflaging this feature is, quite honestly, by covering them up.

Spectacles (Fig. 3.25)

Spectacles nowadays come in all shapes, sizes and colours and should be chosen according to the person's face shape and age. However, if a person does wear spectacles it is important that the choice of hair style is one that complements this feature and does not hinder it. Styles that work best are those that are softly swept away from the face and arranged in soft lines. Any style coming onto the face, or with too much curl around the forehead will

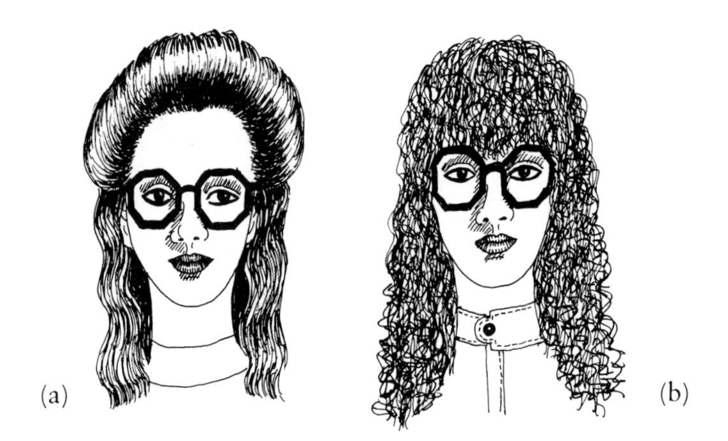

Fig. 3.25 (a) Suitable and (b) unsuitable styles for spectacles.

give the appearance of chaos, and make the whole face area look too muddled.

3.3 THE WAY HAIR GROWS

Hairlines

A hairline is as individual to a person as their face shape, but there are some particular growth patterns around the hairline that seriously affect hair design. It is important that these growth patterns are identified before any final decisions are made on hair styles, or disaster could result, and although hair grows quite quickly, for some poor victim it could seem like forever when they have to wait for a style to grow out.

Widow's peak. This describes when the hair grows into a peak at the centre of the front hairline. It should not be cut too short because it will then stick up.
Cow's lick. This is a very strong growth direction at the front hairline that needs respect as it is impossible to make it lie down flat or indeed go in the opposite direction. This should definitely not be cut too short as it will stick out horizontally. Also, when cutting a fringe, allowances should be made for it.
Receding hairlines. These are when the hair begins to recede back from the front hairline either side of the frontal bone. In these cases the hair should be left to cover this region, and certainly not drawn back off the face.
Nape hairline. This is the hairline at the back of the neck. Care is needed particularly when designing shorter styles because this hairline can grow into a point at the centre of the nape, or into two points, or into three, or sometimes can grow straight across the nape.

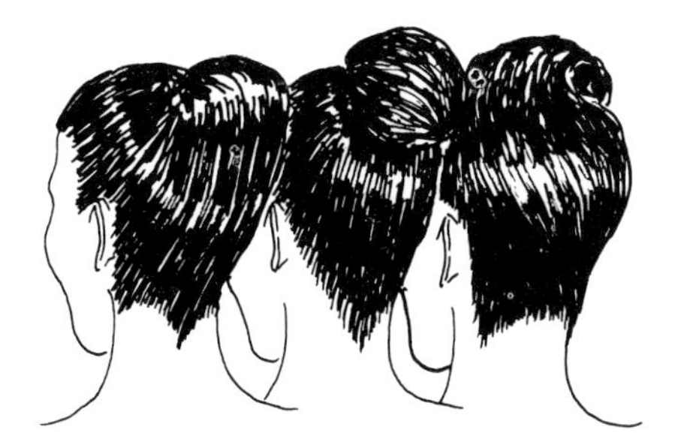

Fig. 3.26 Different shapes of nape hairline.

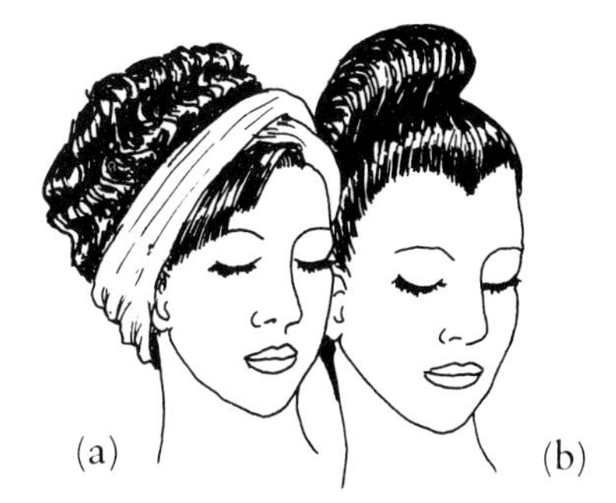

Fig. 3.27 (a) Cow's lick; (b) widow's peak.

Temples and neck. Sometimes the hair can grow from the hairline onto the temples and neck. In these cases it is best to choose styles that cover and disguise the hair rather than choosing styles that require cutting above it.

Crowns

The crown is the point at the top of the head at the back which indicates the direction of hair growth. It has a very strong directional growth that has to be respected. If the hair is cut too short it will stick up stubbornly.

Double crowns. Sometimes there are two crowns situated very close together. This can cause an established growth pattern which nothing can deter. Again, if the hair is cut too short, it will stick out awkwardly.

Partings

Most people have a natural parting where the fall of the hair divides. It is easy to see this if after washing, the hair is loosely combed back off the hairline (Fig. 3.28) and gently pushed down and forward with the hand. The hair will usually part naturally in a particular place. The parting can cause problems if the person wants to change the direction for a hair style. It usually takes a while for the hair to lie in the new direction, and it still tends to part along the natural parting.

Hair type

When choosing suitable hair styles it is best to be realistic. The suitability of any hair style will depend largely on the type, texture and condition of the hair itself. For instance, it would be extremely difficult to achieve a sleek,

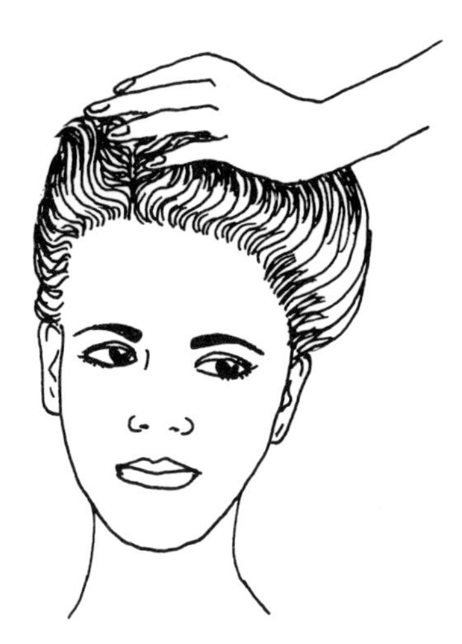

Fig. 3.28 Identifying the natural parting on wet hair.

geometric bob on naturally curly hair, regardless of whether the style might happen to suit the face shape.

3.4 BODY CHARACTERISTICS

When we look at people, we do not confine our gaze to certain isolated bits of them. We automatically view them as a whole, and an assessment of their outlines helps form our impression of them. The same should apply to the hair stylist. When clients come into the salon, stylists do not, or certainly should not, direct their sole attention to the client's head. They, too, should assess the whole body shape, so that the hair style is designed to complement the whole person as well as the head.

Ideally, the head should be able to fit into the body approximately six times, making a total of about seven equal portions. But not everyone is of ideal proportions and there are the long lankies and short tubbies who also want suitable hair styles, so the stylist should be able to offer their expertise to anyone.

If a client is long and thin then the hairdresser should offer styles that add width and certainly no more height or length. Similarly if the client is small and squat, then they should offer styles that increase height and tend to narrow the appearance down, not round, bubbly styles or styles with too much volume as these would only emphasise the squat proportions.

Clothes and fabric designs can also alter the appearance of the build, either in a positive counterbalancing way, or indeed in a negative way that only highlights the build. For instance, vertical stripes will give the impression of lengthening and narrowing, whilst horizontal stripes will give the appearance of widening and shortening. Large prints on a small build will have the same effect as a large print wallpaper in a small room – it will make it appear

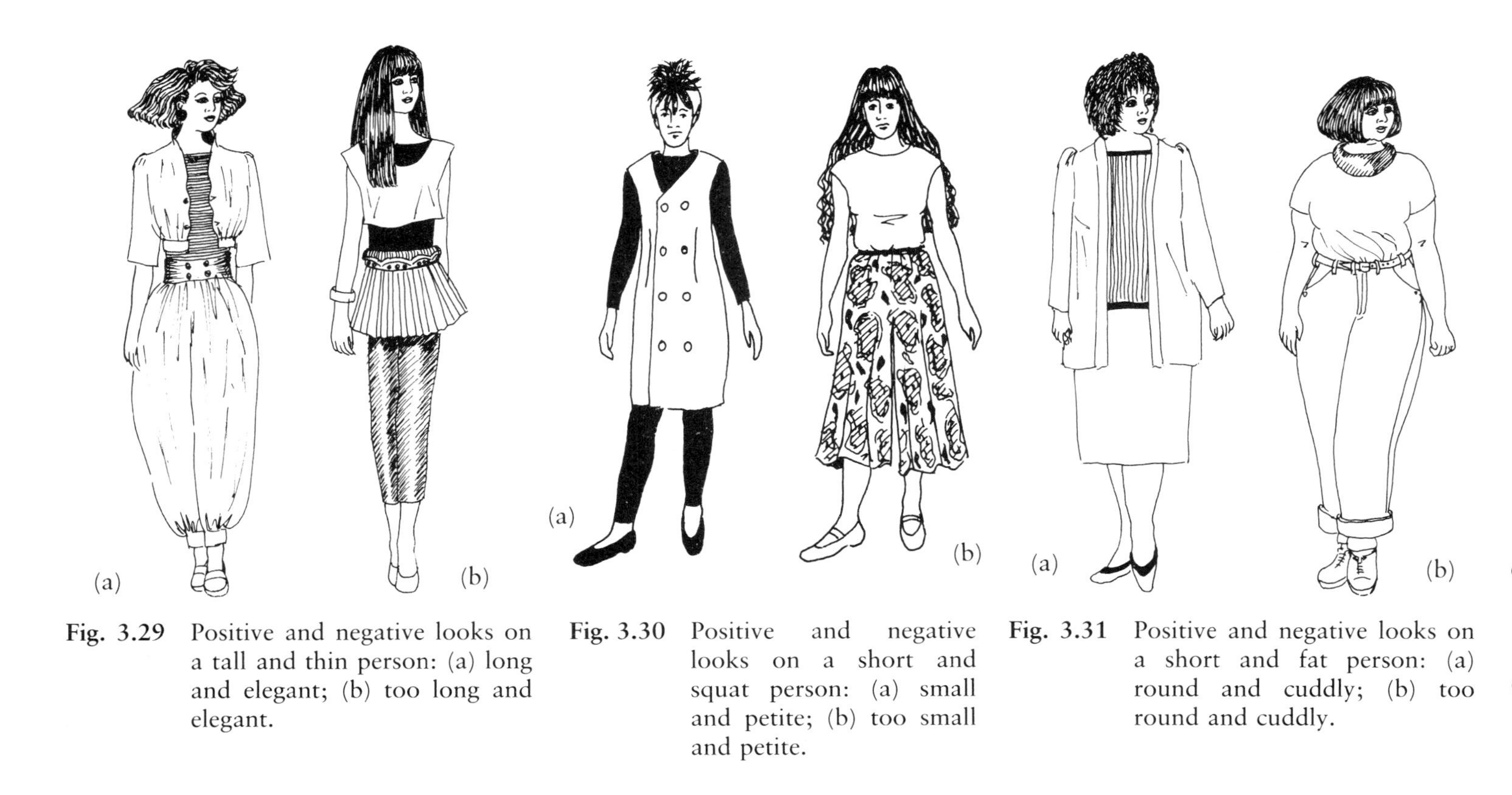

Fig. 3.29 Positive and negative looks on a tall and thin person: (a) long and elegant; (b) too long and elegant.

Fig. 3.30 Positive and negative looks on a short and squat person: (a) small and petite; (b) too small and petite.

Fig. 3.31 Positive and negative looks on a short and fat person: (a) round and cuddly; (b) too round and cuddly.

smaller. It is helpful for hair stylists to know these tips so that they can advise clients if the request should arise.

3.5 IMAGE AND LIFESTYLE

A suitable hair style should fit in with the client's lifestyle. It is not a good choice to give a working person a style that has to be blow-dried every morning, or a person on a limited income a style that needs constant professional care, such as bleaching or colouring.

The image is also important. The client should be observed closely to find a hair style that reflects the right personality. A shrinking violet will not change her reserved personality solely because of the outrageous cut or colouring you offered her. In fact you most likely would never see her again.

The age of the client is another factor to consider, although nowadays, particularly since the 1960s and 70s, styles for different age groups have become much more flexible. There are not really any hard and fast rules. Even so, some styles that are adopted by the younger generation can look strange on an older face, mainly because older faces often do not have the suitable overall shape, and the cut tends to make them look like dolls.

3.6 QUESTIONS ON FEATURES INFLUENCING HAIRDRESSING DESIGN

Complete the following sentences:

(1) The seven basic face shapes are ....
(2) A prominent nose can be minimised by a style that .... but would be emphasised by hairstyles such as ....
(3) A style that adds height without added width at the sides would best suit a client with a .... face shape.
(4) If a client had close-set eyes a suitable style that would appear to set them further apart would be a style where ....
(5) A client with a double chin would best avoid a style that ....
(6) A client with a small forehead would minimise the feature by having a style that ....
(7) Eyes set wide apart would be made to appear closer together with a style that ....
(8) A person with a large round build would best avoid .... type hairstyles.
(9) A client with a long face should choose styles that .... and avoid styles such as ....
(10) A style that added width at the temples, no height, and was narrow at the sides and full at the jawline would best suit a .... face shape.

4

History of Fashion and Hair Styling

Hairdressing is a vital part of the fashion world. It has always been an ingredient that has helped create a new image or look. The best example of this was in the early 1960s when British fashion designer Mary Quant created the mini skirt. The success of Quant was helped by the fact that the prominent hairdresser Vidal Sassoon had designed a hair style specifically to go with the mini. Together they created a new 'androgynous' look on a model called 'Twiggy' that became universally popular. The potential of hairdressing in the fashion world should be taken seriously.

Hairdressing students, like fashion students, should have a basic knowledge of what fashions have gone before. It is only with this knowledge that they can then create new adaptations of old ideas and enter into the innovative world of fashion. The Egyptians are a good starting point when looking at the history of fashion, for although we are aware of cultures that existed before, the ancient Egyptians were sophisticated, and particularly conscious of their appearance. They were also meticulous in recording every occasion and detail through paintings, hieroglyphics (their language of symbols), sculptures and artefacts, so that we have enough information to draw a reasonably clear picture of their fashions, lifestyle and culture. Also we will see that their fashions have exerted a strong influence in later periods.

4.1 ANCIENT EGYPTIANS

The ancient Egyptians were a remarkable race whose culture lasted for over three thousand years BC. Geographically, their location being on the very northern coast of the African continent and practically surrounded by desert, they were inaccessible to intruders and difficult to invade. They had long periods of peace, and with no major outside influence their pattern of life hardly changed. They had sophisticated techniques of clothing technology, and they had master craftsmen in goldsmithing, woodwork, ceramics and the decorative arts. They also had a passion for symmetry and balance. Balance became a basic design element, from their architecture (pyramids), their paintings and sculptures, furniture and bric-a-brac, to the line of their dress, hair styles and headdresses. Everything involving design had to be evenly balanced.

The Egyptians were also obsessed with personal hygiene, which would equal or even surpass today's standards. They removed all body hair with the aid of pumice stone, bathed daily and even washed their hands, arms and necks before and after every meal.

The British Museum has an excellent collection of Egyptian wall paintings, sculptures, mummies, jewellery, toilet articles, such as razors and mirrors, beautifully ornate cosmetic jars, carved combs, wig boxes, etc., which gives an insight into this fascinating race.

Dress

In three thousand years of existence, Egyptian dress hardly changed at all. Women wore a simple sheath falling beneath the arms to the ankles attached by broad straps over one or perhaps both shoulders, more often than not revealing the breasts. They had no inhibitions about nudity, and considering their climate, it was perhaps just as well. Men wore a simple knee-length loin cloth called a 'schenti' which was like a kilt and was attached to the waist by a belt. This seemed to be a common garment for men from workers to the Pharoah or King. The chest was usually bare. Most of the poorer people, such as servants, wore no clothes at all. Dress was considered a luxury reserved for special occasions, and as an opportunity to display wealth.

The popular material used for clothes was linen. In fact, the Egyptians were experts at the weaving of linen, being able to weave finer than is woven today. The actual weave they used was a simple one, but the variations of textures produced was enormous, from sacking to cambric. Wool was also loomed but was not very popular. Garments were usually the colour of the natural white of the flax. Decoration and colour would be added to the dress by means of a wide necklace or collar of brightly coloured beads or precious stones.

Raw materials, such as gold, copper, stone and a vast variety of semi-precious and precious stones were plentiful and were fully employed in garnishing the jewellery the Egyptians seemed so fond of. Colour was very important to the Egyptians, each colour being symbolic of one of the elements. White was considered sacred; yellow/gold represented the flesh of the gods; green represented life and youth; blue represented the skin of Amon (god of air); black was rarely worn. Shoes were rarely worn, and only by the rich on formal occasions in the form of a sandal made from leather or papyrus.

Hairstyles and wigs

Egyptian hair was thick, coarse and dark in colour. The early Egyptians would keep it under control by wearing it in tightly braided plaits, occasionally adding false hair and decorating it with gold or fine glass beads.

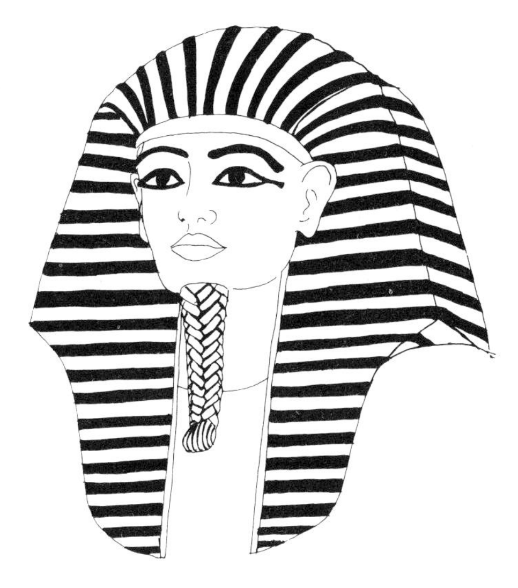

Fig. 4.1 Ancient Egyptian 'nems' headdress.

From wall paintings and sculptures we can see that they had an enormous array of hair styles, and that more often than not these styles would be adorned with some ornamentation – either a band or a headdress.

Later, the Egyptians mastered the art of wig-making, using human hair, occasionally wool or palm leaf fibre and binding it together with beeswax or resin. The construction of the wigs allowed plenty of ventilation, which must have been an essential part of the design when you consider the climate! The wigs also had an adjustable linen drawstring, which could be tied at the temples to secure a comfortable fit. Wigs became very popular and were worn by all those of higher ranking, male and female. The hair was either cropped short underneath or shaven. At first black wigs were popular, but later dyed wigs became fashionable including red, blue and even green! Perched on top of these wigs, particularly at special ceremonies, we can see from drawings, strange bumps. These, true to the Egyptian obsession with personal hygiene, were scented cones of solidified wax, which would gently melt over the wig and body radiating a delicious scent.

The most common image of an Egyptian is probably one of the Pharoah wearing a nems (Fig. 4.1), which is a striped cloth placed round the wig, brought across the ears and tied at the back of the neck, leaving two hanging flaps over the shoulders. On top of this elaborate headdresses would be worn on special ceremonial occasions.

Cosmetics and make-up

Women

Ancient Egyptian women were very beauty-conscious. They spent a long time applying creams and oils to clean and moisten their skin. The legendary

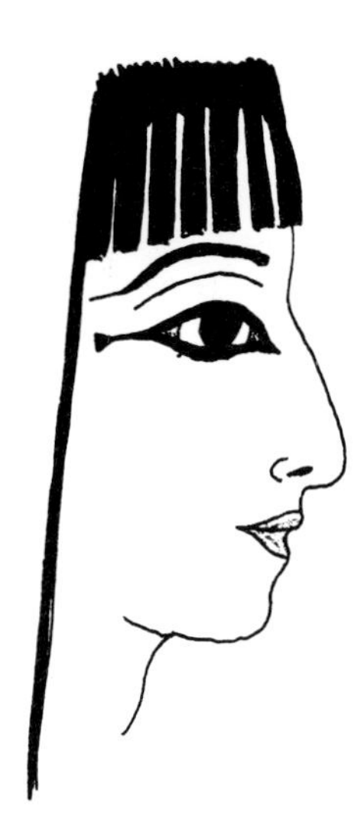

Fig. 4.2 Ancient Egyptian make-up.

Cleopatra, who is well-known for bathing in asses' milk, was trying to combat wrinkles and ageing in an attempt to retain her mortal beauty. Mud packs containing alum were used to rejuvenate the skin, along with honey which was believed to have healing properties. Henna was used to tint the palms of the hands and the soles of the feet a reddish colour.

Perfumes were basically scented oils, made from such ingredients as cinnamon, cardamom, ginger, bitter almonds and peppermint. They were stored in alabaster jars and applied to skin with the aid of small spoons.

Once all the preparation work was completed, the Egyptian 'look', could be completed by applying the characteristic make-up. The main attention was given to the eyes. Eye make-up or kohl, as it was called, was originally applied to both males and females for protection against the glare of the sun, dust, sand, and also flies which carried disease. It was a black or grey-coloured powder usually made up from a concoction of different substances, such as powdered antimony sulphide (a black metallic salt), black manganese oxide, burnt almonds, lead, black oxide of copper, carbon and malachite (a greenish copper ore). It was either mixed with a vegetable oil or moistened to a paste with saliva. Later, galena (a greyish lead ore) was used and became popular. These kohl powders were kept in special small ceramic pots and applied to the eyes with a wooden or ivory stick.

The fashion for this make-up (Fig. 4.2) became quite elaborate, with thick, dark lines around the eye creating a large almond shape – a fashion we will see returning three thousand years later.

On the upper lid, above the kohl line, some women would wear what we would now call eye-shadow, a smear of either blue or green, and sometimes they would wear it below the lower kohl line. The eyebrow would be plucked away, and in its place would be drawn a thick dark line echoing the shape of the eye make-up, or the natural eyebrow would be darkened or thickened

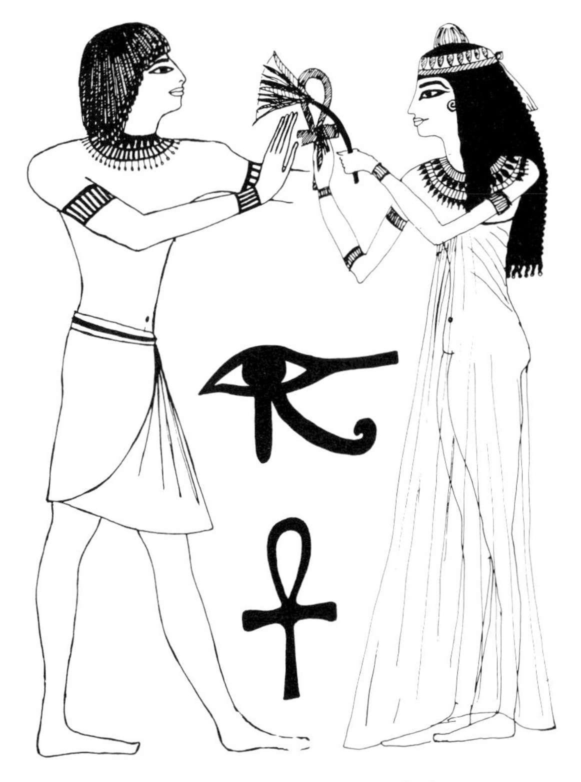

Fig. 4.3 Ancient Egyptian fashions.

with kohl. Powdered red ochre would be rubbed into the cheeks and onto the lips.

Men

Egyptian men would also wear oils and perfumes on their skin. They were clean shaven, but sometimes the higher ranks took to wearing false beards as a symbol of status. The beards were at first made from tightly braided hair and stiffened with beeswax. Later, it became fashionable for the Pharoahs to wear false beards that had been cast out of metals or gold. A curl up at the tip signified their power. Men also wore kohl as protection around the eyes.

4.2 ANCIENT GREEKS

The ancient Greeks were among the greatest founders of European civilisation. They lived in small communities, on mainland Greece and the nearby Mediterranean islands, which grew up over thousands of years and reached their height around 1000 years BC. The Greek philosphers, such as Plato, Socrates and Aristotle laid the foundations of mathematics, the sciences and medicine as well as philosophy. The Greeks also devised the principles of classical architecture, with its idealisation of symmetry and proportion, which are still influencial today. The influence of the Greek culture through language is still seen throughout Europe.

As in Egyptian society, in Greek society we can detect evidence of the existence of what we know today as the 'cycle of fashion', in which old fashions, images and ideas of style have inspired new trends and fashions. The Greeks had a passion for symmetry in design, and they also sought perfection in balance and proportion. There was a cult of physical beauty, and the male human body was considered the ultimate in perfection. Male athletes competed in the first Olympic games and representations of the male form produced exquisite sculptures. Women were also very conscious of their appearance, and created a wonderful array of different hair styles.

Dress

Apart from the early Cretans who favoured more tailored clothes with tight fitting bodices and belts, the ancient Greek style of dress was similar to that of the Egyptians with long, loose-fitting garments, which hardly changed over the years.

The basic item of clothing worn by both men and women was a rectangle of cloth or wool called a 'chiton'. It was worn in a variety of different ways, sometimes wrapped around the body and fastened at one or both shoulders with a pin or brooch, or belted once or twice at the waist, or even belted under the bust. Men usually wore the 'chiton' knee-length, while women wore it ankle-length (Fig. 4.4). On the top of the 'chiton' women would wear a small cloak called a 'peplos'. It is interesting to note here that when ancient Greek statues and artefacts were found during the Renaissance in the 14th to 16th century AD the impression they gave was that the garments were white. When in the cycle of fashion the classical Greek style was revived during the neo-classical period of the late 18th and early 19th century, the new fashions were based on this assumption and white was the fashionable colour. This was in fact wrong. The ancient Greeks actually wore quite colourful and patterned clothes. It was just that time and the elements had taken their toll and the colour and patterns had worn off the statues revealing the white stone underneath.

In warmer weather the men would wear a small cloak, similar to the 'peplos', which would be fastened on one side. It was called a 'chlamys' (Fig. 4.5). In the colder weather they would wear a longer, warmer cloak called a 'himation'. The men were notorious for their splendid armour and helmets, and would enter battle with just a 'chiton' underneath the armour, or they would wear leather tunics studded with metal plaques.

The Greeks were very conscious of personal hygiene. Bathing was very popular and although they did not have soap, they would rub olive oil into their skin and scrape it off along with the dirt with special curved pieces of metal called 'strigils'.

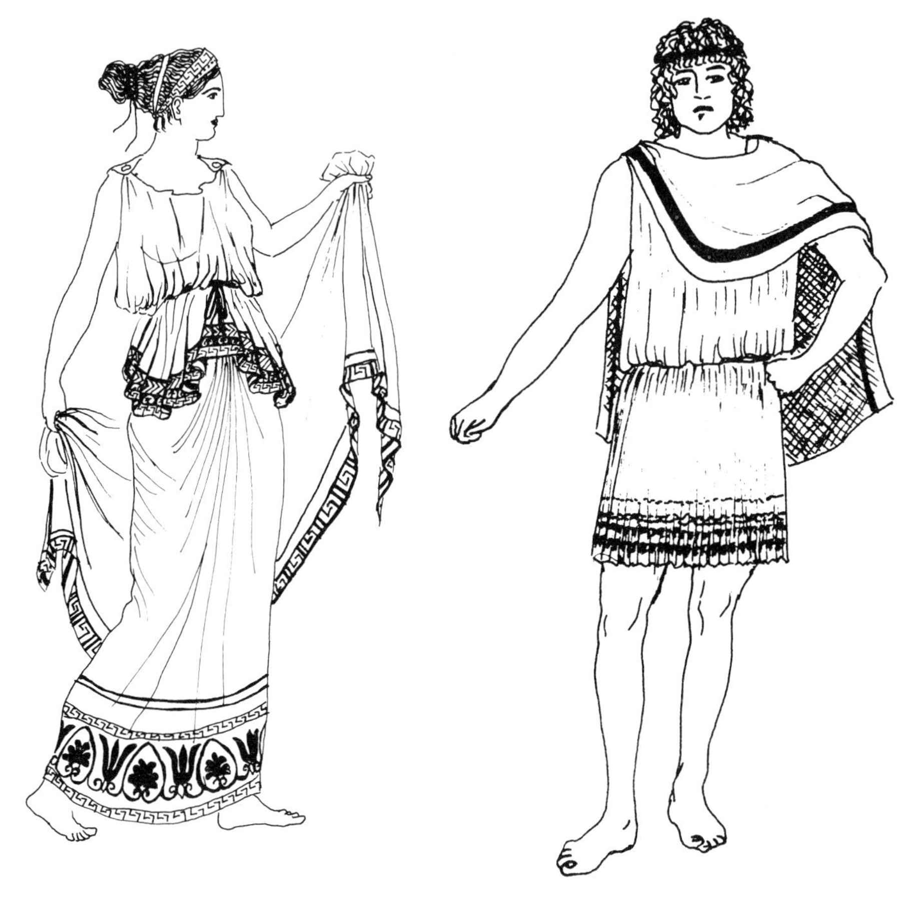

Fig. 4.4 The ancient Greek 'chiton' and 'peplos'.

Fig. 4.5 An ancient Greek man wearing the 'chlamys'.

Hair styles

Women

Early Greeks wore their hair long with a narrow band round the head accentuating its shape. Later, they waved and crimped their hair using various waxes and oils. Their desire for symmetry spread into the dress and certainly into the hair styles. The classical Grecian hair style that remained popular throughout the Roman period and is even around today is parted in the middle, either straight or waved at the sides of the temple and drawn into a chignon at the base of the neck. This style is symmetrical from all angles, front, profile and back.

The classical Greek profile was considered beautiful and a low forehead was also a sign of beauty, so the hair was often dressed onto the forehead in curls and waves, and sometimes false fringes were worn. This straight line

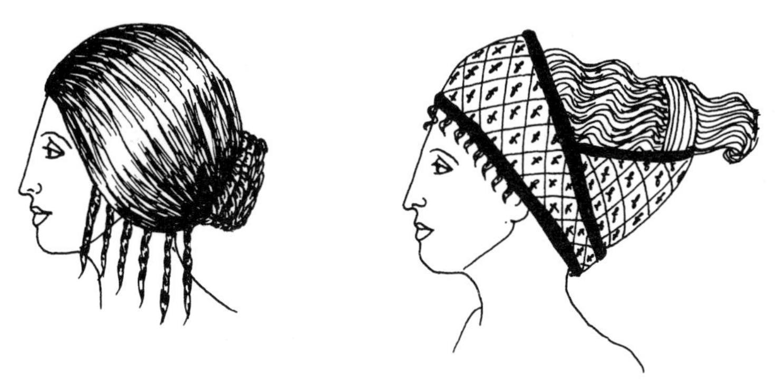

Fig. 4.6 Ancient Greek hair styles.

from the forehead to the tip of the nose can be seen in most Greek sculptures. False hair was also used in other styles that required ringlets or waves hanging down the back. All styles adhered to the basic rule of symmetry (Fig. 4.6).

Flowers, fresh and artificial, were worn in the hair by both men and women in the form of garlands. Young girls wore their hair loose or waved and drawn up into pony-tails, another style we will see revived in the 1950s.

Coloured powders (gold, white and red) as well as dyes were applied to the hair, as blonde hair was popular. Many women suffered sitting in the sun for hours in an attempt to lighten their own hair.

Men

At first men also wore their hair long. Later, they began to bind or twist the hair into coils, fastened at the back in their headbands. They were also mostly bearded. In the latter half of the 4th century BC Alexander the Great introduced the fashion for shaving and wearing shorter hair. This fashion gradually spread in popularity until only officials, philosophers and professional men continued to wear beards.

Men had the first barber shops, which were called 'tonstina' (from tonsure meaning the clipping of hair for religious ceremony), where they could acquire a shave, haircut or massage.

Both men and women wore perfume in their hair.

Cosmetics and make-up

The ancient Greeks were just as fond of cosmetics, oils and waxes as the Egyptians. They took great care over their skin, applying face masks made from meal and asses' milk. Different perfumes were applied to different parts of the body. Early Greeks wore similar make-up to the Egyptians with thick dark lines surrounding the eyes although this fashion was short-lived, being replaced by a more natural look. Women applied a white lead mixture, 'ceruse', to the face to whiten the skin. False eyebrows were fashionable, sometimes stretching across the bridge of the nose. Cheeks and lips were usually reddened with a vegetable tint such as mulberry. Although the more natural look remained popular later, make-up was still worn, but mostly by prostitutes.

4.3 ANCIENT ROMANS

The ancient Roman civilisation had its roots around 700 BC and grew alongside Greek civilisation, at first borrowing much from the Greeks, and later becoming dominant. At first the Romans were ruled by kings until Tarquin the tyrant was banished in 510 BC. Rome then became a republic ruled by the senate and consuls until the first century BC, when dictators (the most famous of whom was Julius Caesar) gradually took over the power of the senate. The first Roman emperor was Augustus Caesar, who in the early years AD founded a great empire which lasted until the Dark Ages (about AD 400).

The Roman Empire stretched throughout Europe, North Africa and the Middle East, and the civilising influence of the Romans shaped Western culture and dominated it for many centuries. Whatever was fashionable in Rome was fashionable everywhere. The period after the downfall of Rome is known as the Dark Ages because the civilising influence of Rome was lost for a while. The Renaissance (or rebirth) was the name given to the time when Roman culture was rediscovered, starting in the 14th century. At this time attempts were made to copy Roman civilisation exactly. Roman culture dominated again (with Greek) as late as the 19th century during the neo-classical period, when as we shall see later in this chapter, fashions again revived those of the ancients.

The Romans did not share the Greek obsession with the beauty of the male human body, but instead saw women as the pinnacle of beauty. Men aspired to dignity rather than beauty. The Romans also did not share the Greek attitude to nudity. Many women followed the traditions of the matrons of the Roman Republic and were extremely modest. They considered exposing the body uncouth and paramount to sexual enticement. These women would cover their heads when in public for decency. However, during the time of the Empire, personality cults grew up round the emperors and their families, who took the lead in more opulent and decadent fashions.

Dress (Fig. 4.7)

The early form of Roman dress was a simple, linen loin cloth, but later, the basic form of Roman garment for men became the 'toga'. This was worn as a symbol of Roman citizenship, and members of the Roman senate were distinguished by the right to wear a purple border to their 'togas'. The 'toga' consisted of a semi-circle or rectangle of natural wool or cloth, draped over

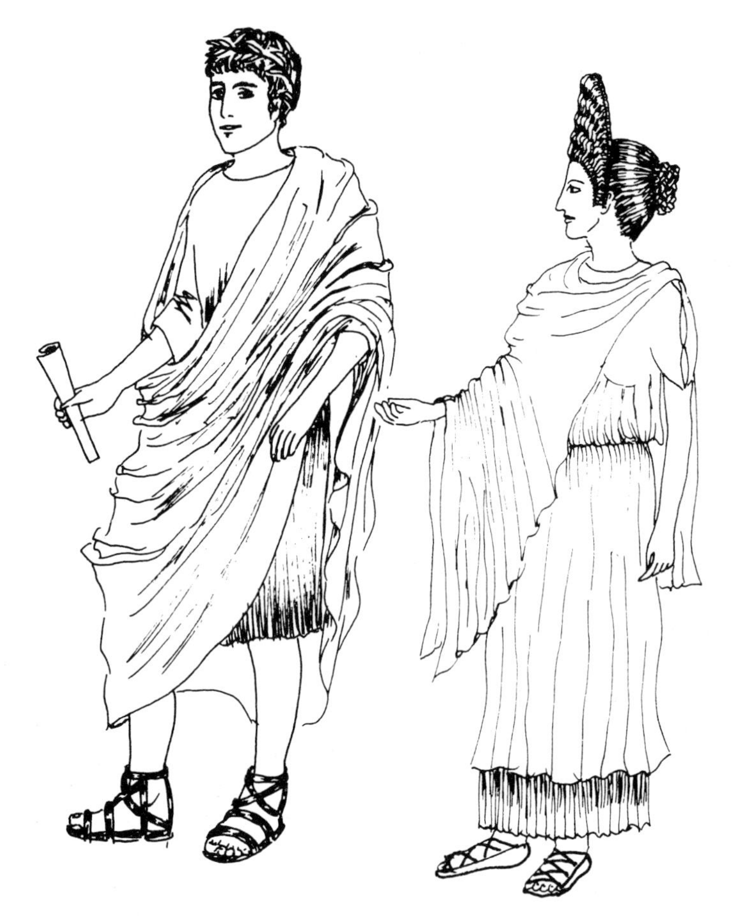

Fig. 4.7 Male and female Roman fashions.

and around the body (in a similar way to the Greek 'himation') and usually one end would be draped over one arm. Underneath the 'toga' would be worn a 'tunica', which was a simple linen tunic, similar to the Greek 'chiton'. It was usually knee-length and belted at the waist.

Early female Roman dress was similar to the male dress except for a 'strophium', which was a bust bodice worn under the 'tunica'. Women wore their 'tunicas' much longer than the men. The female version of the 'toga' was the 'stola', which was a more fitted robe, but still loosely draped. It was usually belted beneath the breast and also at the waist. It also had sleeves and fell in deep folds to the ankles. In colder weather over this they would wear a huge, hooded cloak called a 'palla'.

Men usually wore white, whereas women's dress was much more brightly coloured: yellow, blue and red. The most common materials used were natural wool, linen or cotton, but also silk by those who could afford it.

Footwear consisted of simple leather sandals which later became more elaborate. Knee-high leather boots were worn in the armies during the colder weather. Indoors, women wore delicate slippers (called socci), which were usually studded with precious stones, depending on the wealth of their owners.

Hair styles

Women

To begin with, the female Roman hair styles followed the simple symmetrical styles of the Greeks, but soon they became more elaborate and grossly unbalanced, resulting in some hideous creations that were quite ugly and not at all flattering to the shape of the head. One of the most characteristic of these styles was the 'orbis', which consisted of several bands of curls projected from the forehead and dressed over crescent-shaped wire frames. The rest of the hair would be drawn back into a pony-tail or a coiled bun at the back. (This very unbalanced shape we can see revived again in the 18th century with the extremities of the Georgian wig fashions and even in the 20th century with the back-combed beehives of the 1950s.) These elaborate styles required a lot of time and also the assistance of a 'tonstrix' (female hairdresser), who would arrange the desired curls with the aid of an ample supply of false hair, heated tongs and lotions.

Hairdressing became a passion among Roman women and hair styles became numerous and changed rapidly. Wealthy Roman women were very fashion-conscious even to the extent that bald female portrait busts have been found, presumably so that different sculptured hair styles could be placed on to keep up with the fashion.

Blonde hair was very fashionable. Many women experimented with bleaches on their hair, sometimes with disastrous results, but women mainly took to wearing blonde wigs that had been made with hair taken from slave girls from the north (Germany). Yellow wigs were, by law, worn by prostitutes, but a fashionable trend for them was instigated by the notorious Messalina, wife of the Emperor Claudius, who was reputed to frequent brothels on her nightly jaunts.

Precious stones and metals were used in hair ornamentation in the form of hair pins and combs.

Men

Early Roman men were bearded and wore their hair quite long. During the Republic beards were still worn but it became fashionable for the hair to be worn short and simply. Later, from about 200 BC, the fashion for shaving grew and only scholars and philosophers wore beards so as to emulate the learned appearance of the Greeks. The hair was worn reasonably short, but well oiled, waxed or curled with the aid of heated tongs. The style was usually dressed forward. This was an attempt to disguise those who were balding, as baldness was considered a deformity. Many obnoxious lotions were concocted to try to prevent it. False hairpieces were also used, being glued to the scalp and carefully coiffured. Julius Caesar adopted the wearing of a crown of laurel, as an honorary wreath for either military or academic achievement, but it also acted as an adequate disguise for his balding condition. Barber shops or parlours were common in Rome and also acted as good meeting places for men to discuss business or topical issues. The more wealthy had their hairdressing services done at home by special slaves. The popularity of blonde hair affected men too, although they did not go as far as dyeing it or adorning blonde wigs, but the wealthy did apply gold dust to lighten it.

Emperor Hadrian, in the second century AD, reintroduced the fashion for beards. His was said to disguise unsightly warts on his chin, but the trend became very popular. This fashion was also subjected to extensive grooming; the beards were oiled and curled into elaborate shapes.

Cosmetics and make-up

Women

Wealthy Roman women spent several hours every day preparing themselves, with the help of numerous slaves, in bodily decoration. They too, like the

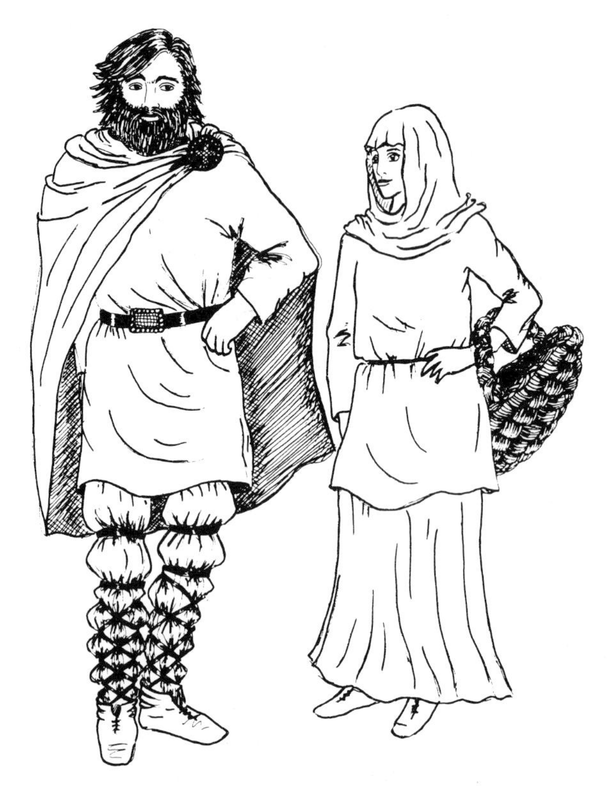

Fig. 4.8 Anglo-Saxon fashions.

Greeks, were fastidious about their personal cleanliness and bathed at least once or more often twice or three times a day. The body hair was removed with pumice stone, except the eyebrows which were tweezered into shape. Depilatories were also experimented with. The skin was kept soft and supple with the various oils that were massaged into it. Face packs containing flour and asses' milk, or honey and wine dregs were used in order to rejuvenate tired, wrinkled skin. Both men and women wore perfumes which must have been quite spicy, made from flowers, scented woods and spices.

Make-up became more obvious and colourful than in Greek society. It took on more of the appearance of the Greek prostitutes. The Roman make-up consisted of a very pale complexion, which the Roman women achieved by painting their faces, like the Greek women, with a white lead powder (ceruse) obtained from Greece. The eyes were outlined and the eyebrows made more pronounced by using kohl (obtained from Egypt), stibnite (a black powdered ore of antimony), lead or soot. The cheeks were rouged using iron oxide, red lead or carmine (which is extracted from the cochineal insect) and the lips were also painted red with carmine.

Men

Roman men also spent a great deal of time over their appearance. They were particularly fond of perfumes and lotions to grace their bodies. They also wore make-up for special occasions, but not to the extent that the women wore it.

4.4 ANGLO-SAXONS

The Romans ruled most of Britain for about 400 years, and during this time fashions and hair styles emulated those worn in Rome. The next great shift in fashions in Britain occurred after the departure of the Romans around 410 AD and the disintegration of the Roman Empire. Britain was invaded by a succession of barbaric tribes from the European continent, chief amongst whom were the Anglo-Saxons from Germany.

Information concerning the fashions, hair styles and life-styles during the Dark Ages is thin. One of the best references we have is the Bayeux Tapestry which recorded events preceding, during and after the Battle of Hastings in 1066. The tapestry was completed in 1092, and gives us a good insight into what was worn at the time. Also, illuminated manuscripts and brass rubbings offer additional information about the fashions and styles.

Dress (Fig. 4.8)

The fashions of the Anglo-Saxons were very primitive in comparison to Roman dress. A tunic was the basic garment roughly made from wool or flax and sometimes, according to the season, a second tunic would be worn over the first. The men wore their tunics knee-length and in colder weather they would wear woollen leggings and leather shoes or thick wads of wool that were strapped up around the calf of the leg.

On top of their tunics they wore cloaks, which would be fastened at one or both shoulders by a clasp or brooch. Women would wear their tunics ankle-length and over the top they would wear a 'mantle', a form of short cloak sometimes with a hood attached. They too wore woollen leggings and shoes.

Although dress was extremely simple, the Anglo-Saxons loved to wear jewellery in the form of buckles, brooches, necklaces and rings. Noblemen and women could afford jewellery made from gold and semi-precious stones, while the poorer wore jewellery made from bronze and melted glass.

Hair styles

Hair styles were based on practicality. Long hair was worn for the extra warmth to the head. Sometimes it would be plaited. More often than not the head would be hooded. Men wore their hair shorter and in colder weather took to wearing small, cone-shaped, woollen hats. Most men were bearded.

There is not enough evidence to tell whether Anglo-Saxon women wore any oils, perfumes or make-up. Certainly the Roman Britons must have worn similar cosmetics and make-up to their counterparts in Rome, but the contrast in life styles was extreme and make-up and toiletries seem out of context to this primitive, basic life style.

4.5 THE MEDIEVAL PERIOD

The Viking invasions of Britain, during the late 10th and early 11th centuries, had little effect on the customs and fashions of the people. The next strong influence came from the Normans from France. Their conquest of Britain was completed by the death of Harold at the Battle of Hastings in 1066. The Bayeux Tapestry gives us a useful insight into what the Normans wore as well as the Anglo-Saxons.

Dress (Fig. 4.9)

Women

Early Norman dress consisted of variations to the basic tunic. It was worn sometimes short to the knees, or longer to the ankles. Sometimes a longer tunic was worn with a shorter outer tunic on top, called a 'dalmatic', which had sleeves and tended to emphasise the cuff. The material was either wool or linen, and the Normans liked to decorate their garments with a border design. These tunics were usually worn with a belt around the waist. The hood had become a separate piece of clothing and was worn like a very loose balaclava with a shoulder cape.

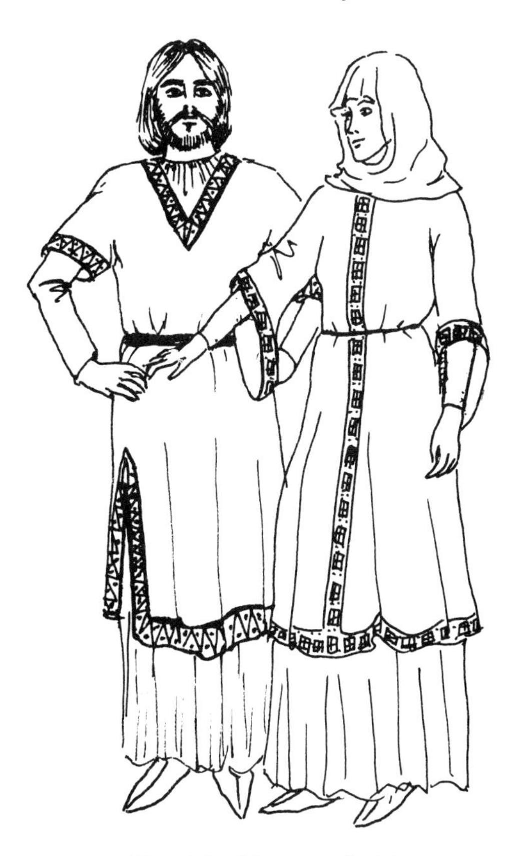

Fig. 4.9 Norman fashions.

Later, around 1100 AD, a new style appeared for the noblewoman. A tighter-fitting bodice to the hips was worn (replacing the outer tunic) with a fuller skirt which fell in folds to the feet or even longer, forming a train. Suddenly the female figure was revealed. This early form of corseting was achieved by tight lacing at the back. The sleeves became a feature about this time, being worn tight to the elbow, then belling out into very wide cuffs. These cuffs grew to incredible widths, even so far as to be hanging to the ground (Fig. 4.10).

Another fashion that started about this time was the wearing of a 'girdle', which was a leather band worn over the gown, wrapped around the waist, and fastened on the hips with silken tassels attached in the front and left hanging down to the feet.

Men

Early Norman men wore their tunics at knee-length and either wore woollen breeches or hose. Breeches were ankle-length trousers corded at the top for support. On top of these sometimes would be worn leg bandages, which were strips of cloth bound round the legs in spirals or criss-cross. Hose were like

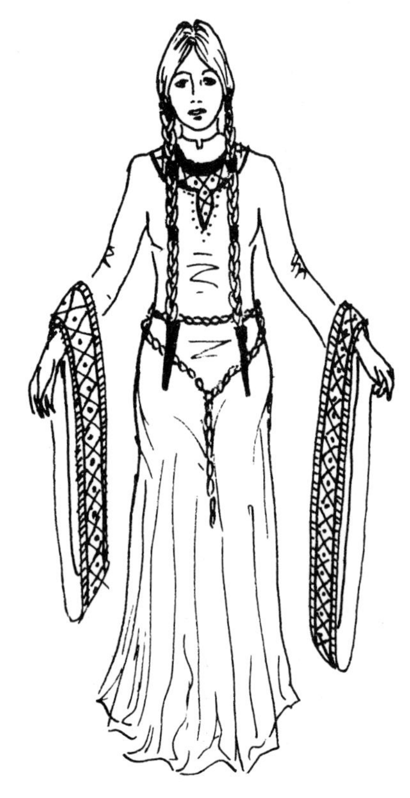

Fig. 4.10 Female fashions of the 12th century – the figure begins to be revealed.

knee-length stockings. The other variation of dress was the longer under-tunic worn under a shorter outer-tunic. Both styles were belted. Later, the hose extended to mid-thigh and was worn pulled over the breeches.

Both sexes would wear leather sandals (if they could afford them) or thick woollen pads on the feet.

Hair styles and headdresses

Women

Women began to display their hair again in the 12th century, being very proud of their long tresses. Plaits became very popular and grew to enormous lengths, even to the ground. All sorts of schemes and devices were used to make the hair appear abundant. Extensions were plaited in silk, gold and silver sheaths; false hair was also used. The ends of the plaits were weighted with heavy ornaments to hold them straight (see Fig. 4.10). Sometimes four plaits were worn, two hung over the shoulders in the front and two behind.

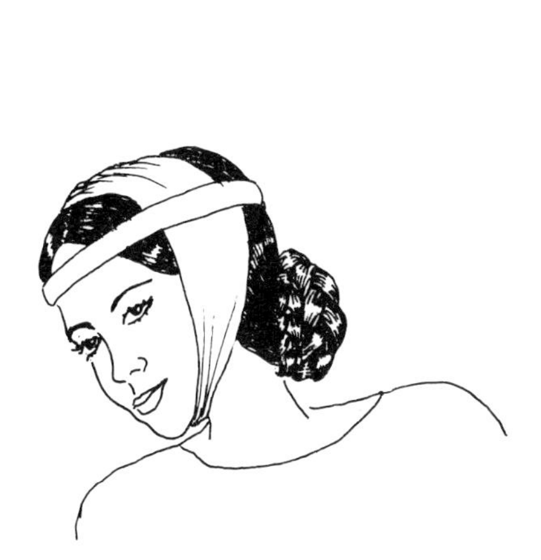

Fig. 4.11 'Barbette' and 'fillet'.

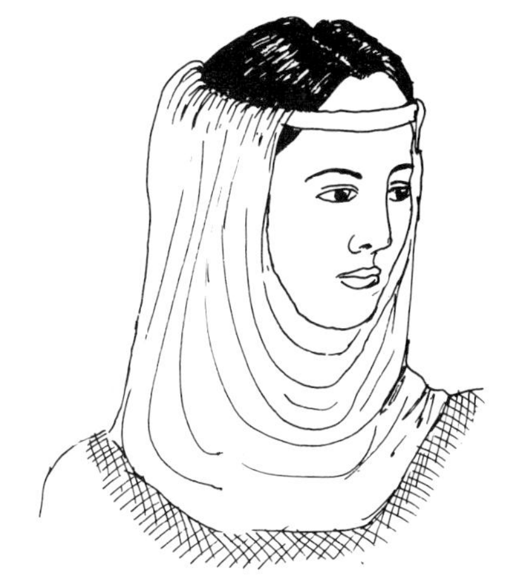

Fig. 4.12 Variation on the 'wimple' – the 'Gorget'.

Long plaits were popular until about 1170, when the fashion required shorter plaits wrapped round the head and secured at the front.

Earlier fashions in headdresses saw a simple veil being held in place by a band of gold worn around the head. Later, towards the late 12th century, a band of material was worn under the chin and pinned around the head. It was known as the 'barbette' and became the basis for headdresses until the early 14th century. At this particular time the 'barbette' was usually worn with a 'fillet' (see Fig. 4.11), which was a band of cloth that was worn around the head over the top of the 'barbette'.

Another important form of headwear that stayed popular for about 200 years was the 'wimple'. It consisted of a length of linen that was draped under the chin, obscuring the throat and pinned to the hair at the crown. It was usually worn with a veil. Later, it was sometimes worn without a veil and the ends would be tucked into the coiled hair at the temples. It was then called a 'gorget' (see Fig. 4.12).

Blonde hair was fashionable and women would sit for endless hours in the sun with their hair stretched out in an attempt to lighten it. Later, saffron dyes were used to lighten the hair.

Men

Early Norman men wore their hair long and were usually bearded. Later, the hair was worn shorter and they were clean shaven, although this fashion was short-lived. Beards and moustaches were soon worn again, but this time they were kept neatly trimmed. Men wore several forms of hats, one of the most common still being the hood, worn as a separate garment with a shoulder cape. Other common forms of headwear were the 'phrygian' hat, which was a sort of pointed beret, and the 'coif' (see Fig. 4.13). The 'coif' was a small linen hood that sat snugly on the head and had flaps that covered the ears. It tied under the chin. This headwear stayed fashionable for both sexes until the

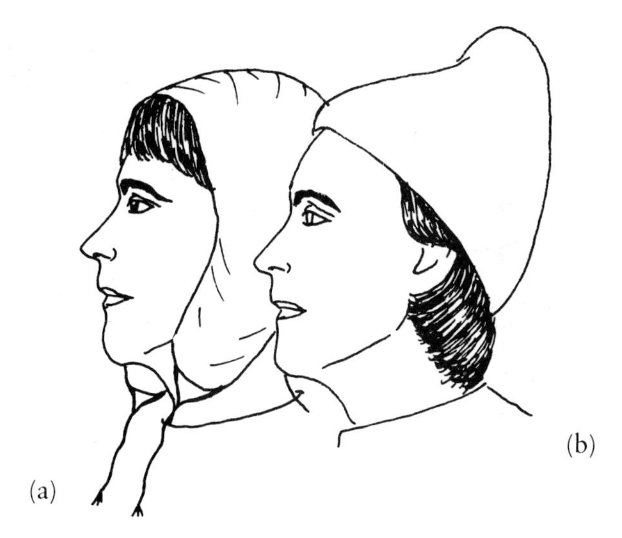

Fig. 4.13 (a) 'Coif'; (b) 'phrygian' hat.

Tudor period of the 16th century. Wide-brimmed hats were worn when travelling, usually over a 'coif'.

13TH AND 14TH CENTURY

The next great stimulus to changing fashions came in the late 14th century, as Britain began to recover from the devastation of the plague. Emancipation from the feudal system also brought newly acquired wealth, although humble, to the poor, and this led to a revived interest in dress.

Dress

Women

During the late 14th century the slender waist became a desirable feature following on from earlier trends (see Fig. 4.10). The result was the introduction of the corset (a lace-up version) to acquire this desirable shape. This was, perhaps, an innocent development but it was to become the curse of women throughout history, periodically developing into extremes and grossly distorting the figure. The gown was still the basic garment in the 13th and early 14th centuries, but the wearing of the girdle disappeared and was replaced by a sort of sleeveless, sideless tunic worn over the gown, called a 'cyclas'. This extra garment subsequently made the 'mantle' cloak unpopular (Fig. 4.14). The 'cyclas' then disappeared with the development of the tighter-fitting gowns of the late 14th century. Materials became heavier – in particular velvet, which was popular. Another feature about this time was the

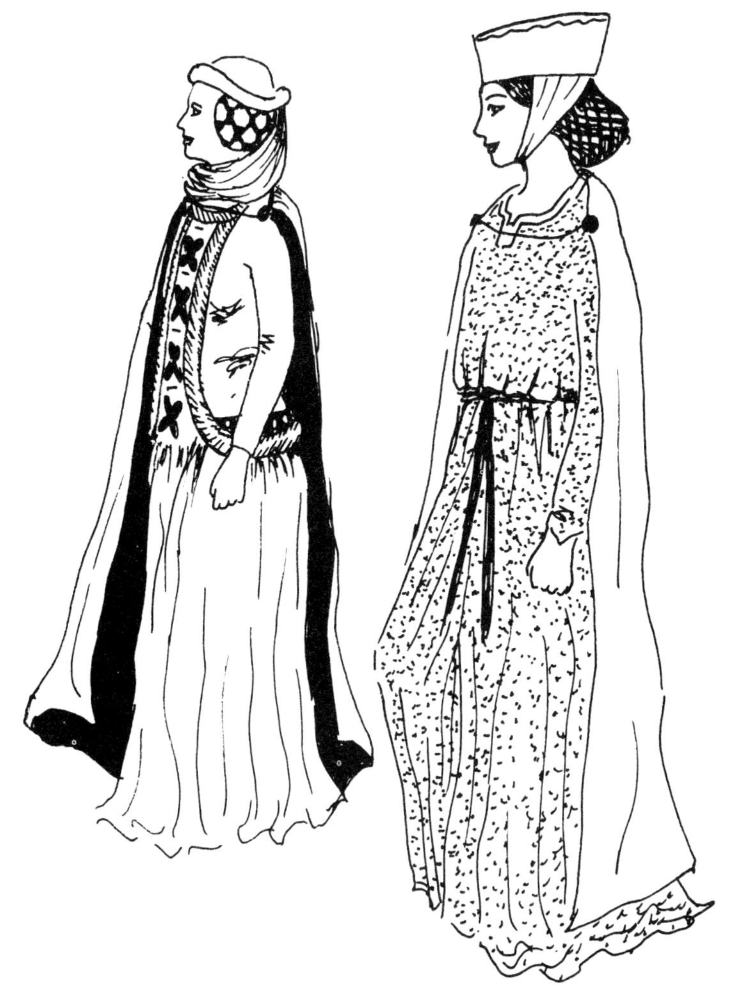

Fig. 4.14 Gown and mantle cloak of the 13th century (in foreground) replaced by the popular 'cyclas'.

wearing of long strips of material that were attached to the elbow, called 'tippets' (see Fig. 4.15).

Men

One of the important adaptations to dress for men was the 'surcote' or super tunic, worn over the basic under tunic. It was adapted from the tabards worn by the crusading knights. First it was sleeveless, being slit at least to the waist, but later it adopted sleeves. The 13th century saw the passion for Gothic architecture, and the long tall spires started to be echoed in the shape of the dress. Pointed shoes became very fashionable, although they were to reach their peak more towards the 15th century (see Fig. 4.15).

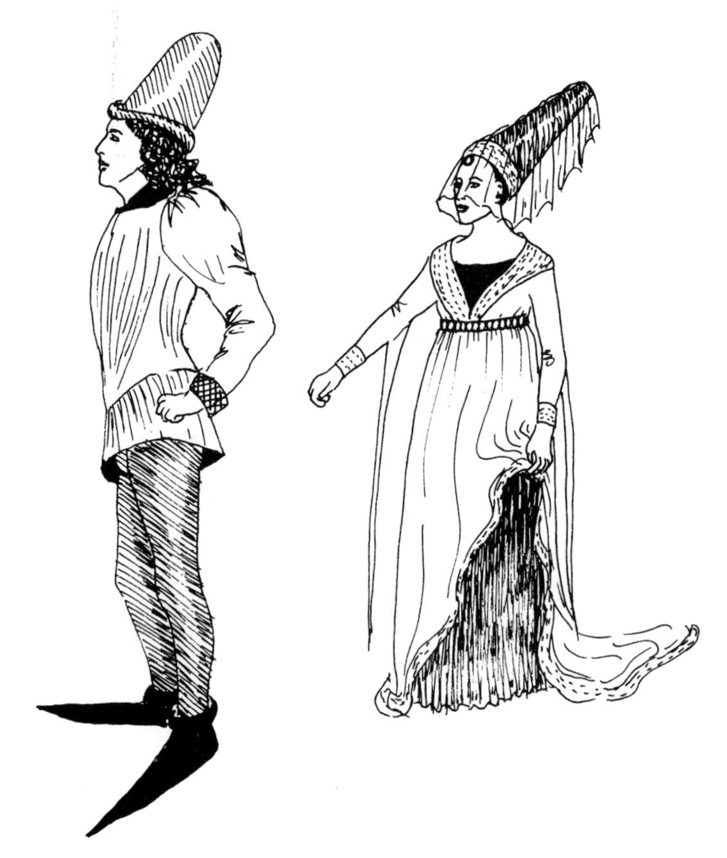

Fig. 4.15 14th century female fashions showing the trend for 'tippets' and the male 'gothic' style of dress.

A feature that was characteristic of the 14th Century was 'dagged edges', which was when the hem and sleeves of the tunic were cut to give a jagged effect (see Fig. 4.16).

The late 14th century saw the disappearance of the 'surcote' and the introduction of the 'cotehardie', a tighter fitting, shorter over-tunic that required the wearing of a full hose (similar to tights).

Hair styles and headdresses

Women

A form of headwear emerged in the 13th century which was usually worn with the 'barbette' and became popular with most women until the late 14th century. It was the 'crespine', a sort of caul net that encased the coiled or plaited hair at the nape of the neck (Fig. 4.17). It was an important feature as it became the basis for many headdresses in the succeeding centuries and has stayed with us throughout history, reappearing periodically: Victorian caul nets; 1940s snoods; a version of it is even around today in the slightly

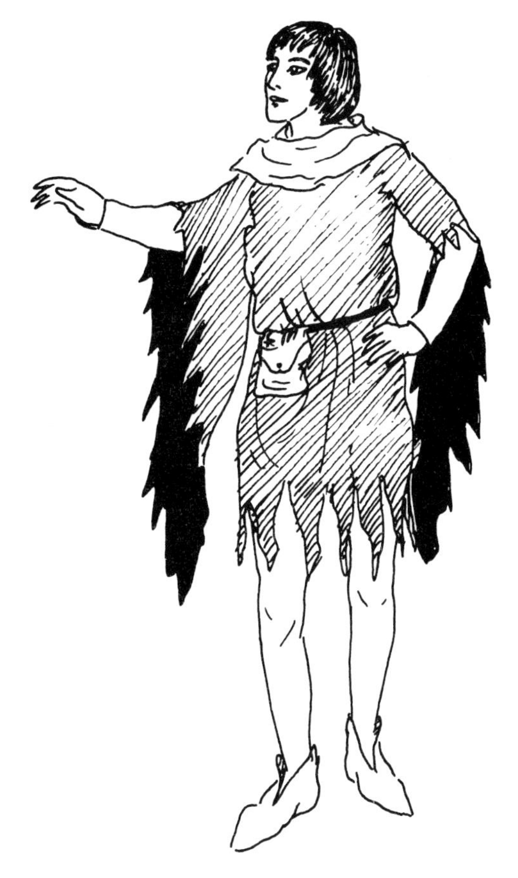

Fig. 4.16 'Dagged edges'.

smaller, circular nets used to envelope buns, etc. The tendency to cover the head more became apparent in these centuries, and it was not until the 16th century (Elizabethan period) that the head was exposed again.

Another characteristic style of the 14th century was the wearing of a 'crespine' with two long plaits worn at either side of the head. The 'circlet' was another popular headdress of the 14th century. This was an open-work metal casing worn either side of the face and joined by a decorated metal band or fillet worn around the forehead (Fig. 4.18). The hair would be plaited and folded into the casing. The 'cushion' headdress consisted of a padded roll worn over the hairnet or 'crespine' with the hair coiled at the temples (Fig. 4.19). An important fashionable detail of the late 14th century was the trend for women to shave or pluck their hairline back to attain the very fashionable high forehead that had become so desirable. This continued until the end of the 15th century.

Men

During the 13th century men wore their hair in a very basic bob style, a style that has been revived many times throughout history but worn more by

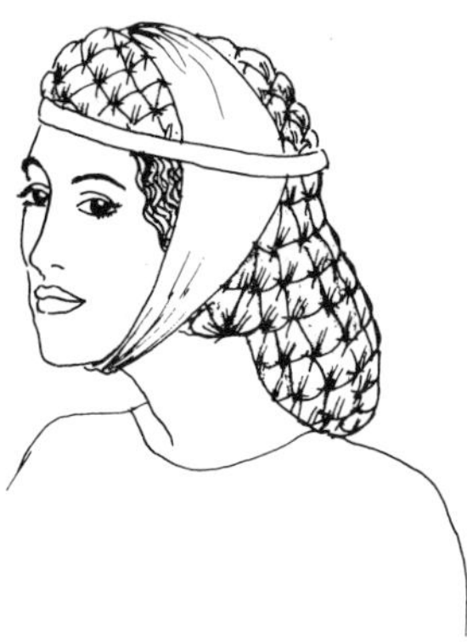

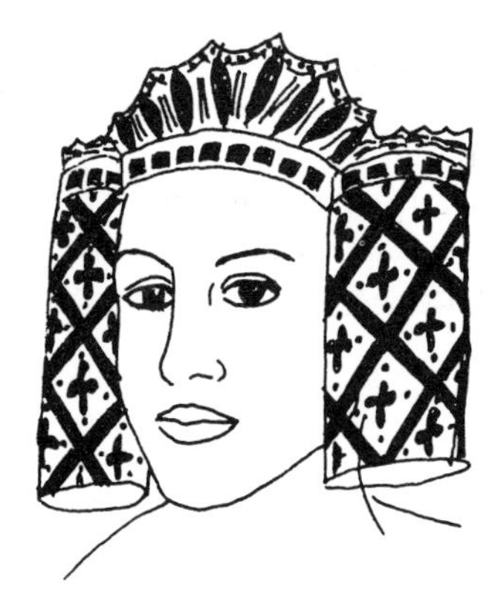

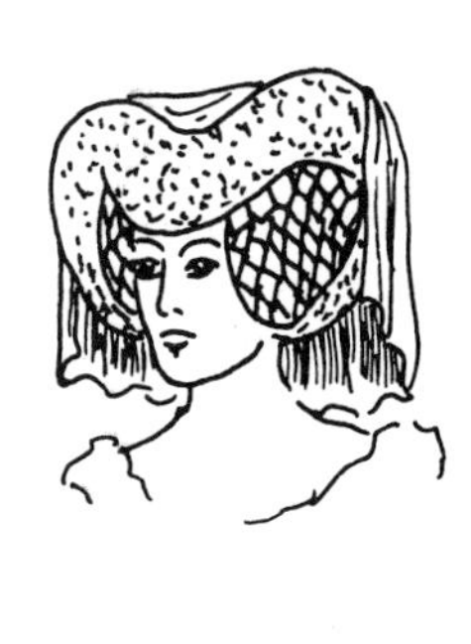

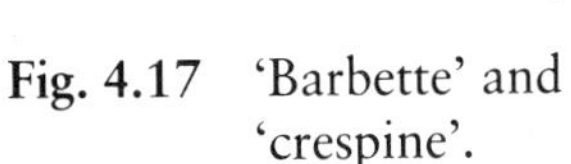

Fig. 4.17 'Barbette' and 'crespine'.

Fig. 4.18 'Circlet' headdress.

Fig. 4.19 'Cushion' headdress.

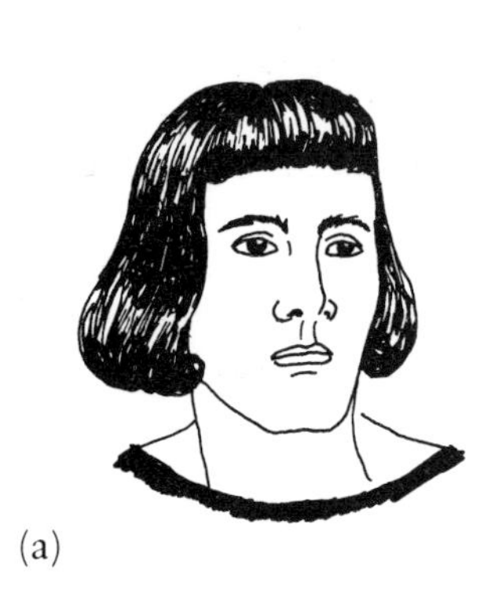

(a)

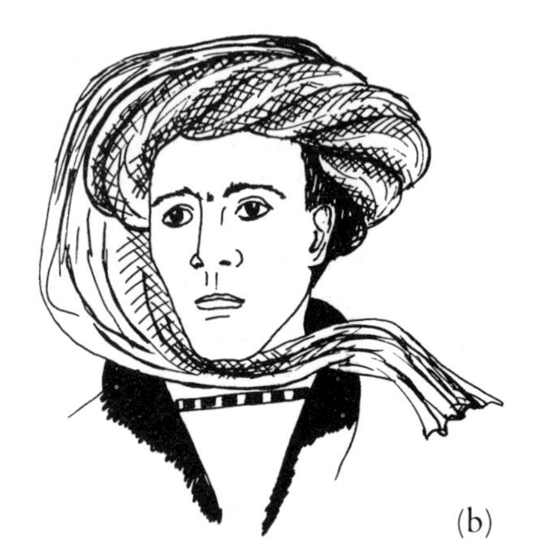

(b)

Fig. 4.20 (a) Typical 13th century men's bob hair style; (b) the 'chaperon' hat.

women. It was parted in the middle just above the forehead and the sides were dressed into loose waves and rolled under at the jaw line. The most popular form of hat for men was the 'chaperon', which was made from cloth into a circular padded roll with folds of material attached to the top. These would be either hanging down loose or gathered up round the face, keeping the hat secure (Fig. 4.20).

Cosmetics and make-up

Women

Paintings and portraits from this period indicate that women in the 13th and 14th centuries preferred a very clean, sometimes virginal look. The skin was usually portrayed as delicate white and totally unblemished with the appearance of porcelain. The eyes were left natural. The only indication of make-up was rouge on the lips.

The fashion for plucking eyebrows was popular, although unlike the ancient Egyptians these women did not replace the eyebrow with a drawn line. Considering the raised hairline, the face must have appeared extremely bare (see Fig. 4.23).

Men

The same paintings and portraits show no signs of men wearing any form of make-up or any obvious alteration to their facial features.

4.6 15TH CENTURY AND THE EARLY TUDOR PERIOD

The 15th century saw a great struggle by a succession of short-lived kings to establish themselves on the throne. This culminated in the Wars of the Roses, finally won by Henry Tudor, who was crowned Henry VII in 1485. He established the Tudor dynasty which lasted until the death of Elizabeth I in 1603.

The Tudor period was one of comparative stability in government, in which increasing prosperity was reflected in renewed interest in fashion. The Tudor monarchs displayed a fondness of extravagance in dress fuelled by the arrival of exotic materials from the New World.

Early 15th century headdresses

Women

The fashion for headdresses that had started in the 14th century became more elaborate in the early 15th century. Hair was hidden as it was considered improper for married and mature women to reveal it. Only young girls were allowed to do so. Women were expected to cover their hair with a drape, headdress or bonnet. Headdresses became extensions of the costume, creating an overall style or image.

Early 15th century headdresses still adhered to the vertical line of design, with such creations as the 'horned' headdress, which consisted of a wire structure in the shape of cow horns with a veil draped between them, or the 'chimney-pot' headdress, which is self-explanatory in description. This was usually worn with a 'barbette' (Fig. 4.21). A popular headdress of the period was the 'hennin' or 'steeple' headdress, which was a sort of truncated cone and had a veil attached that gently fell down onto the forehead and draped around the head (Fig. 4.22).

One of the most elaborate headdresses must have been the 'butterfly', a heavily embroidered flower-pot shaped hat with two wires attached

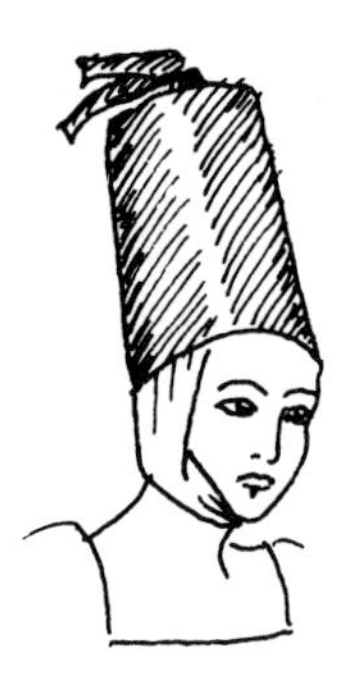

Fig. 4.21 'Chimney-pot' headdress worn with a 'barbette'.

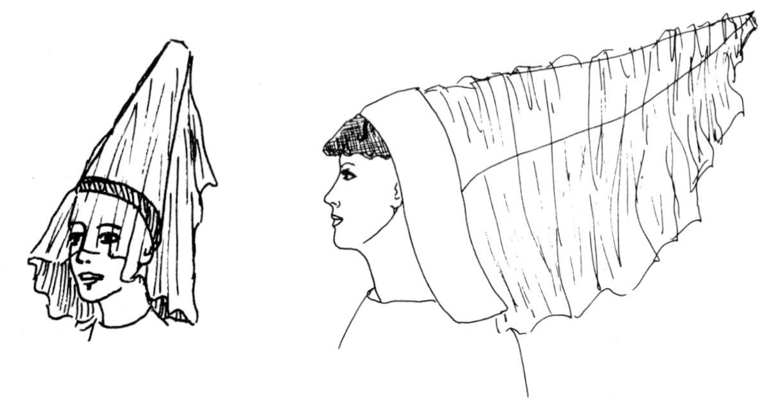

Fig. 4.22 Variations of the 'hennin' or 'steeple' headdress.

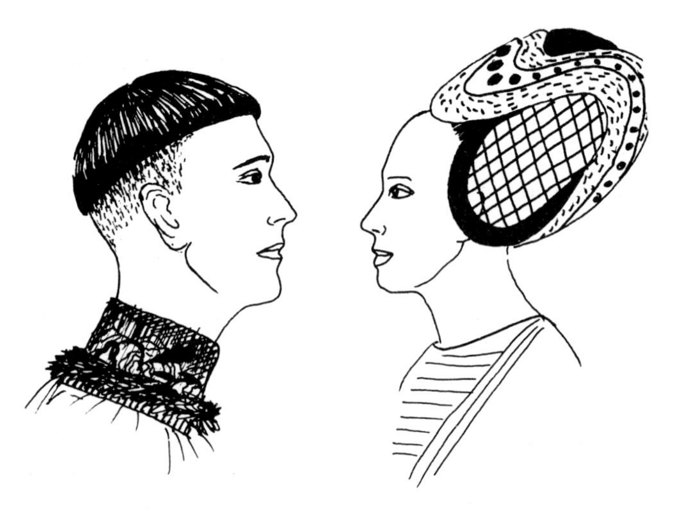

Fig. 4.23 Late 14th century and early 15th century hair fashions showing the plucked hairline and male 'bowl' crop.

supporting a stiff gauzy veil that simulated butterfly wings. The veil was attached to the front of the hat or to the hair.

Men

The most important style for men which appeared about 1410 and stayed popular for about fifty years was the bowl crop, which suggests that the barber put a bowl on to the head and cut around it. In fact that is just what it looked like (Fig. 4.23). The back hairline was shaved to the level of the ears and the rest of the hair radiated from a centre point with the ends curled under, like a crude pageboy style. Men were usually clean shaven.

Tudor dress

During the 15th century dress hardly changed from the kirtle and gown until the Tudor period, when an interest in dress and style took on a serious vein, and suddenly money could be spent on clothes by those who could afford them. This was the period of voyages and discoveries, which meant that new, more luxurious materials became available. Costly fabrics, fur and heavy jewellery, and the thick embroidered fabrics helped give the costumes that required stiffness. For the first time in the history of fashion functional purposes of dress gave way to decorative effect. The fashionable costumes that were created completely ignored the shape of the body underneath. Artificial shapes required uncomfortable distortion to fit the shoulders, waists, stomachs and hips, and a number of devices such as corseting, padding, wiring, bejewelling and moulding were employed.

Early Tudor styles still had a strong French influence (first established in the Norman period) and one of the major changes was in the actual line of dresses and headdresses, which had up to this period been steadily getting more vertical in design. Suddenly the line began to be more horizontal. The low, square Tudor buildings that started to appear were reflected in the horizontal lines of the costumes. The line and shape of shoes also changed. For so long they had been very pointed, now suddenly they became square-toed and broad.

Men still wore the doublet and hose although the fabrics used were of much richer quality.

One of the major changes to dress in the late 15th century for both men and women was brought about by the German influence on style. In particular, slashing (which was the art of cutting slits in the material of the garments and pulling through the lining underneath) became universally popular with the fashion-conscious Tudors by 1500, along with the use of richly embroidered and brightly patterned materials. The most favourite materials used were velvet and satin. Also popular were fur trimmings on almost every garment. The most popular furs that were used were lynx, wolf and sable. The poorer people wore simpler, more practical clothes made of rough woollen cloth or coarse cotton. Children wore miniature versions of their parents' clothes.

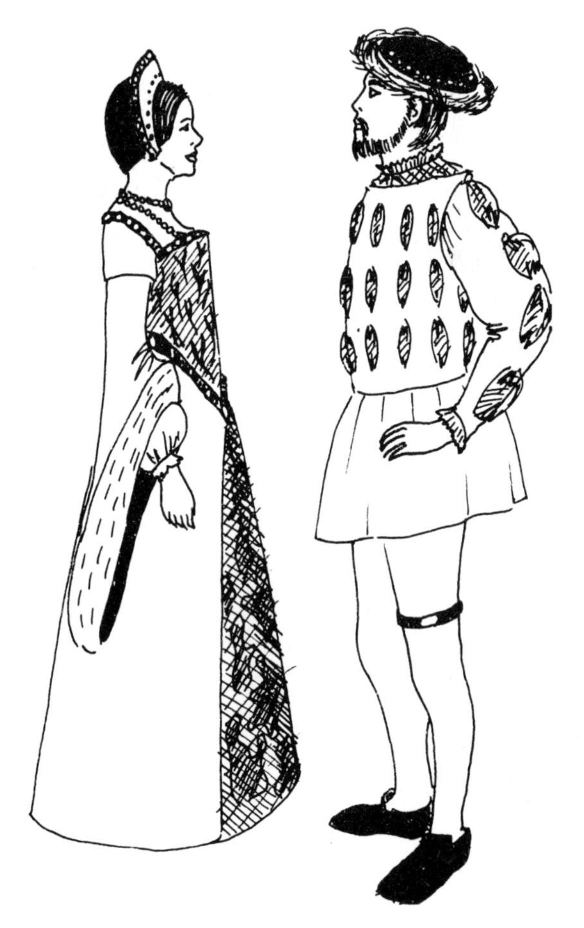

Fig. 4.24 Horizontal line of Tudor dress depicting female 'French hood' and the popular trend for slashing.

Women

The line of the dress was squarish and broad. The kirtle and gown were still worn, although later it became popular to discard the gown and just wear the kirtle. The skirt became a smooth cone shape, without folds or drapery, worn with just a stiff petticoat underneath. A new style of bodice appeared about 1493. It was still tight-fitting with a low, square neck but began to have a wide V opening down the front to the waist, or even below, emphasising the petite waist. The sleeves became wide and usually were bell-shaped (see Fig. 4.24).

Men

Henry VIII had a rich wardrobe of fashionable, highly decorative clothes which included expensive and lavish materials. He enjoyed wearing rich,

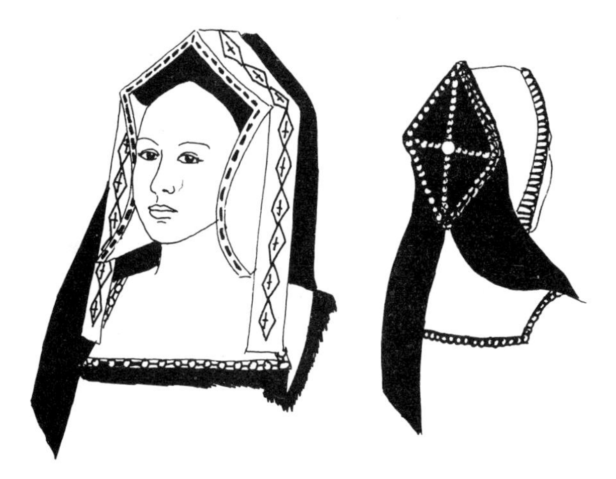

Fig. 4.25 'Split gable' headdress.

colourful garments and set the pace in court for the fashion-conscious. The fashion still included the doublet, which was worn over a shirt, usually satin or silk, which would be drawn through the slashings (see Fig. 4.24). The shoulders would be padded and the sleeves full. Short breeches would be worn, which had an opening at the front revealing the codpiece. Over this would be worn a gown or cloak, which fitted loosely over the shoulders and fell full to the knees or ankles. The gown was usually edged with fur. A hose or tights would be worn and broad-toed shoes, called 'duck-bill', which were made from leather, velvet or silk. These too were often slashed and studded with jewels.

Tudor headdresses

The change in design from vertical to horizontal affected the headdresses as well, and one of the first Tudor headdresses created on this line was the 'bonnet'. It derived from the 'hennin' headdress, but now adopted a round crown, front bands and long side pieces that hung down. This eventually developed into the popular 'gable' headdress which strongly resembled the Tudor roofs. A variation of the 'gable' that later developed into a popular headdress was the 'split gable' (see Fig. 4.25) where the cloth hanging down the back was split in two and one of the lengths was turned up and pinned on the top. The 'French hood' was another favourite (see Fig. 4.24), particularly of Anne Boleyn (the second wife of Henry VIII). The hood exposed some of the front hair, which was usually worn parted in the middle. Widows and elderly women still took to wearing the 'wimple' (a fashion carried over from the 14th century) with the gable hood.

Caps were also fashionable for women as well as for men and were particularly favoured by Catherine Parr (sixth wife of Henry VIII).

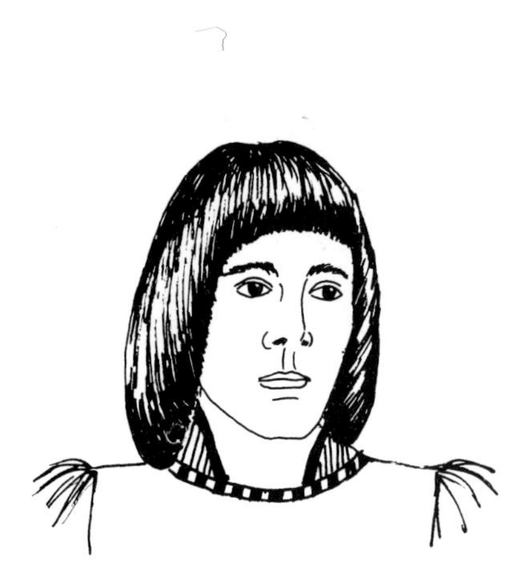

Fig. 4.26 The 'polled' hair style.

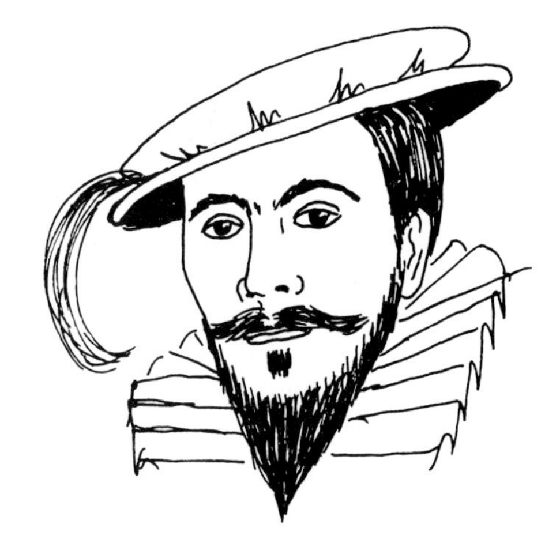

Fig. 4.27 The Spanish influence on Tudor fashions.

Men

The earlier 'bowl crop' style developed into more of a bob style by the 1520s and was called the 'polled' (Fig. 4.26) Henry VIII also set the fashion for beards again. Hair styles came under Spanish influence during the reign of Mary Tudor, who was married to Philip II of Spain. By 1550 the pointed Spanish moustache and beard were universally worn, along with shorter hair styles that were parted in the middle and flattened (see Fig. 4.27).

Hats and caps were worn by practically everyone, and there was a wonderful selection of styles. Undercaps or 'coifs' were worn indoors. Wigs of white or yellow silk attached to berets were occasionally worn tilted on the head.

Cosmetics and make-up

The look was still very natural and virginal. The high forehead was still quite fashionable but not so fierce as it had been in the early 16th century. Eyebrows were plucked and lips rouged.

Men started to blacken their eyebrows to make them more pronounced.

4.7 ELIZABETHAN PERIOD – LATE 16TH CENTURY

Dress

One of the most characteristic features of Elizabethan dress was the ruff. It was derived from the drawstring tops of the shirts or undergarments of the earlier Tudor period, that were pulled tight round the neck, resulting in a

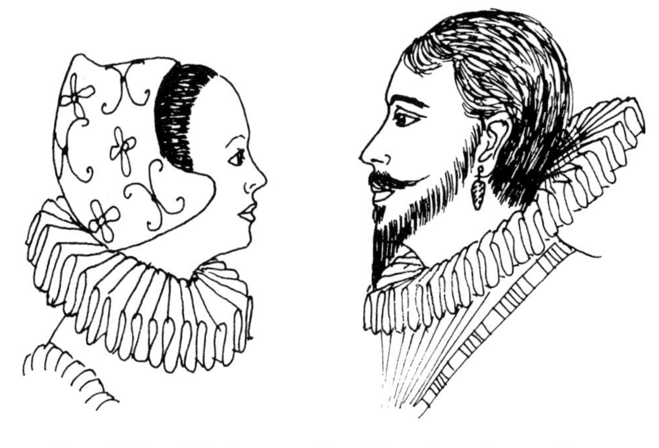

Fig. 4.28 Medium ruff stiffened with starch.

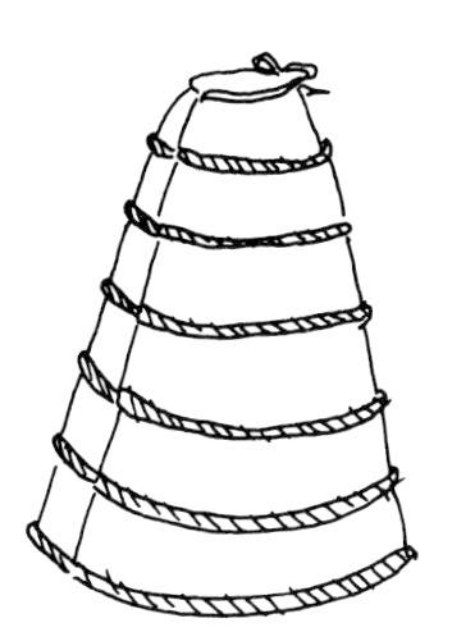

Fig. 4.29 Spanish 'farthingale'.

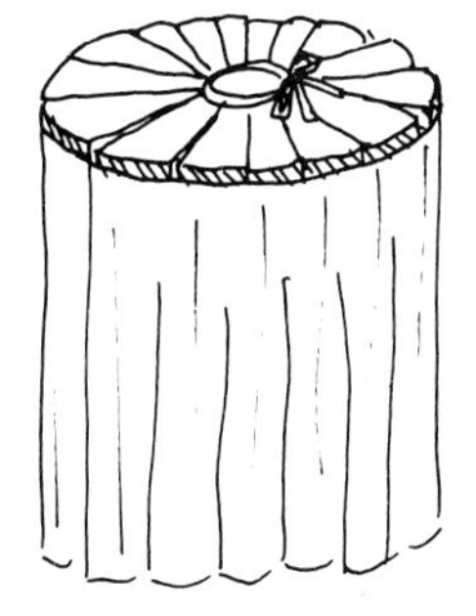

Fig. 4.30 French 'farthingale'.

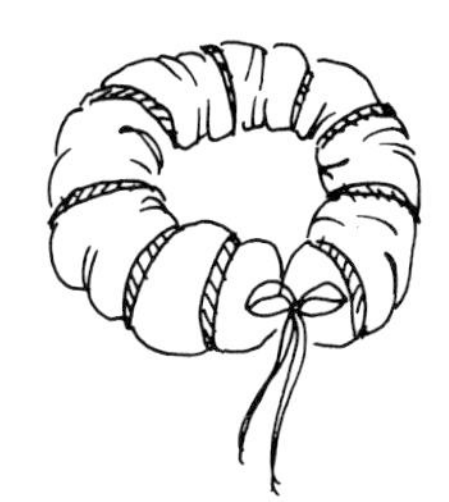

Fig. 4.31 'Roll' or 'bum roll'.

heavily gathered top visible above the doublet or kirtle. The ruffs were made from cambric and were basically of two types. The medium ruff was stiffened by using starch (a new invention from Holland) and was closed all the way round the neck (Fig. 4.28). The cartwheel ruff was a larger collar, supported by a hidden wire frame (see Fig. 4.35 below).

Another characteristic feature of the Elizabethan period was the 'farthingale'. The first came from Spain and was worn about 1545. It consisted of a hooped under–skirt in the shape of a bell made from wire, wool or whalebone (Fig. 4.29). Later, the French 'farthingale' became popular. It was also made of wire or whalebone. The framework extended out from the waist and hips and fell to the ankles resulting in a cylindrical shape (Fig. 4.30). The middle ranks of society favoured another, less extreme, version of the 'farthingale', known as the 'roll' or sometimes 'bum roll'. It consisted of a padded roll of cloth in the shape of a sausage being tied round the waist and joined together in the front (Fig. 4.31). Boned bodices made of whalebone were worn to acquire the desired shape (Fig. 4.32).

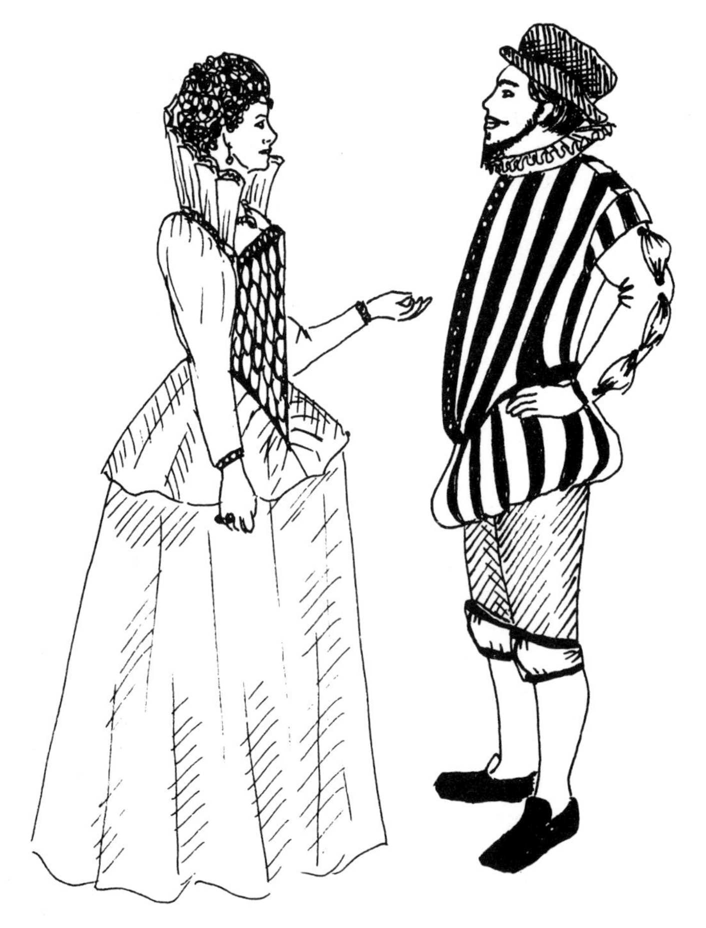

Fig. 4.32 Elizabethan dress depicting boned corsets and French 'farthingale', worn by women to acquire the desired shape, and the male 'peascod body'.

Rules were laid down for dress in court. For example, the colour crimson could only be worn by persons of royal blood. Shoulder sashes were a popular feature worn by both men and women, but only white sashes could be worn by the Queen. Commoners could wear velvet but only on the sleeves of their dress.

There was no major change to the style of dress in the latter half of the century, except that sleeves became tighter, and they were usually detachable, being joined by hidden buttons. Women began to wear drawers from the 16th century. They were a type of trouser tied at the waist and reaching down to the knee, where they were fastened to the stockings by garters. They were usually made from cotton, but silk and brocade were also used. Woollen stockings became popular with the invention of the first knitting machine in 1589, and both women and men wore them.

Men

The fashion of dress did not change a great deal in the Elizabethan period, but the style of dress did. The Spanish influence brought the trend of padding the breeches with bombast (a concoction of rags, flock, horsehair, cotton and even bran). The doublet was padded extensively too, so that the waist amongst all this padding must have appeared slender.

A new introduction to the doublet was a version of the Dutch 'peascod body', which was additional padding placed at the point of the waist. This resulted in the illusion of an extended belly that overhung the girdle (see Fig. 4.32).

Hair styles and headdresses

Elizabeth I made it respectable for women to reveal their whole head of hair (something that had not been done since the 12th century). She totally dominated fashion, and as she had naturally red hair fashionable women sought to dye their own hair using concoctions of sulphur, lead, quicklime and water. This was not always successful and wigs quickly became an alternative. The Queen owned many herself, particularly as she got older and her own hair became very thin and sparse.

The hair fashions and headdresses were all designed to sweep up off the neck and add height to complement the heavily, starched, up-standing collars. The hair was usually frizzed or tightly curled, and was either closely cropped and brushed upwards into a bristle effect with the aid of gum (a similar style to those adopted in the 1950s and 1980s) or had a centre parting with the hair rolled back at the temples over rolls or pads. Later these pads were developed into wire frames called 'palisadoes', and the aim was to make the hair appear abundant. An Italian version was similar except that the two crescent-shaped pads met in the middle of the forehead and a pearl or jewel hung onto the forehead. The hair at the back was coiled into the nape, and small curls ('hairlocks') would be worn just in front of the ears. There were many varieties of headdresses worn. A popular one was the 'atlifet', which was a version of the 'French hood' but with a wired edge (see Fig. 4.33). Another was the 'taffeta pipkin', a sort of stiffened beret with a rim. This was usually worn with a 'snood', a similar net to the crespine worn in the 13th century that encased the hair at the back of the neck. The hat was sometimes decorated with feathers worn in the brim. Soft materials, such as silk, velvet, taffeta, leather, felt and sometimes beaver were the most popular for hats. Older women continued to wear the 'French hood' (Fig. 4.34).

Men

Headwear was very popular both outside and in the home. The materials used – silks and velvets – came from abroad, causing excessive importing, which was very damaging to the English cloth manufacturing industry. In 1565 Queen Elizabeth I issued an Act of Parliament that halted further

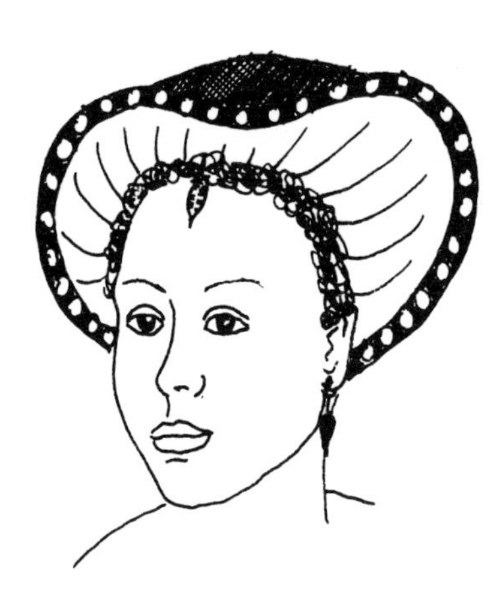

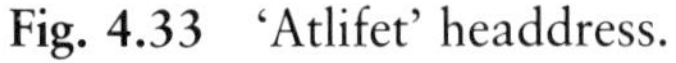

Fig. 4.33 'Atlifet' headdress.

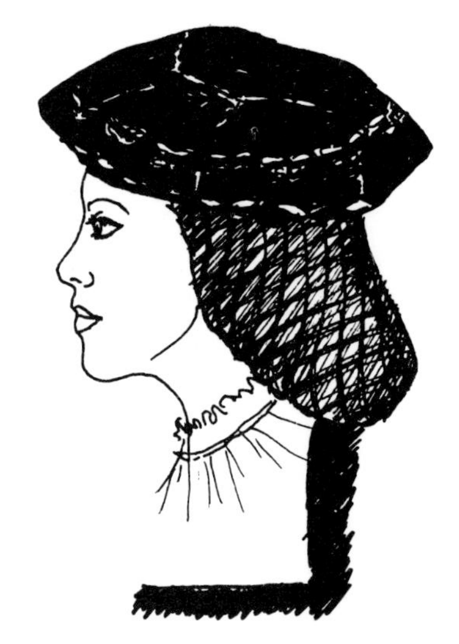

Fig. 4.34 'Tafetta pipkin'.

importing and ordered every male over the age of six years and on an income of under £40 per year to wear a woollen cap (that had been manufactured in England) on Sundays and holy days. The popularity for velvet and silk hats was hard to deter and the Act was constantly disobeyed to such an extent that it had to be reintroduced in 1597.

Men's hair styles varied. Some wore it curly and long, decked with pearls and precious stones, while others wore it short, parted in the middle and accompanied by a full beard and moustache. In fact, beards were extremely popular and men became incredibly vain about them, powdering, waving, scenting and even dyeing them. It also became fashionable for men to wear an earring in one ear. This fashion stemmed from the explorers and navigators on expeditions who found that it was the safest place to carry the precious stones they found on their travels.

Cosmetics and make-up

Make-up was widely used, certainly more than it had been since Roman times. The basic colours of the make-up were red and white to complement the fashionable red hair. The face was whitened with a lead mixture that was painted onto the skin. This withered the eyelashes and eyebrows, and also, because of the lack of dental hygiene, discoloured and rotted the teeth relatively quickly. The Queen herself suffered. Powdered borax, which was not so harmful to the skin, was sometimes used instead of lead.

Whitened skin was a symbol of refinement and many women tried different inventions to achieve it. One concoction involved gathering dew-drenched peach blossom at dawn. This then had to be crushed with oil of almonds by the light of the moon. Another was to wash one's face in one's own urine or to wash with rose water and wine.

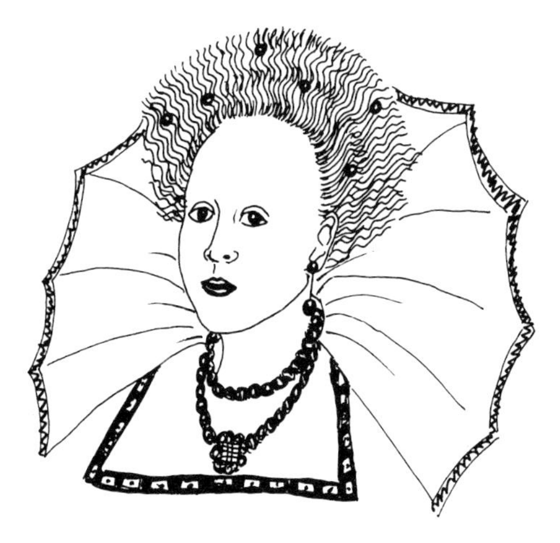

Fig. 4.35 Elizabethan look with 'cartwheel' ruff.

The cheeks were rouged with a mixture of ochre and mercuric sulphides, and the lips rouged with either cochineal blended with gum arabic, egg white and fig milk, or ground alabaster or plaster of Paris mixed to a paste with a vegetable dye. The Queen's use of make-up (Fig. 4.35) became more vibrant as she grew older. She would even vermilion her nose! Face paints, although very popular with women, were disapproved of by the Church. Another fashion was for wearing patches. Originally, small black silk patches were worn on the temple as a cure for toothache. The contrast of black against the extreme white became fashionable, and developed into different shapes that were worn over the face, shoulders and bosom.

4.8 17TH CENTURY – THE STUART PERIOD

After the death of Elizabeth I in 1603, James I (her cousin) came to the throne and began the reign of the Stuarts. James I was already king of Scotland and he therefore brought about the unification of Scotland with England. The Stuarts had a very different style of rule from the Tudors, and they quickly became unpopular. A struggle ensued between the Stuarts and parliament, which was seeking power for itself. Another source of conflict was the difference between the puritans, who led strict lives in accordance with a narrow set of religious principles, and the supporters of the Church of England with the King at its head. The puritans organised an army known as the roundheads with Oliver Cromwell as its leader. They challenged the second Stuart king, Charles I, and his supporters known as the cavaliers in a civil war, which ended in 1649 with the execution of the king. There followed a brief interlude with Oliver Cromwell and the puritans in power before Charles II restored the Stuart monarchy in 1658.

The conflict between puritans and cavaliers was reflected in their styles of dress. The cavaliers favoured lavish, colourful clothes and admired elegance,

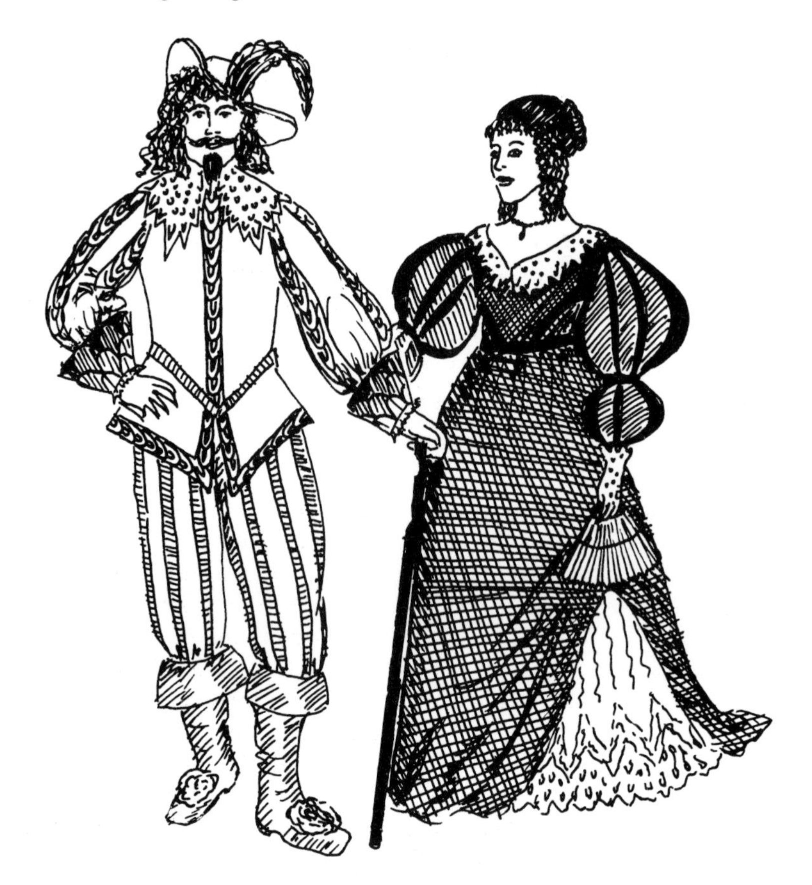

Fig. 4.36 Stuart fashions.

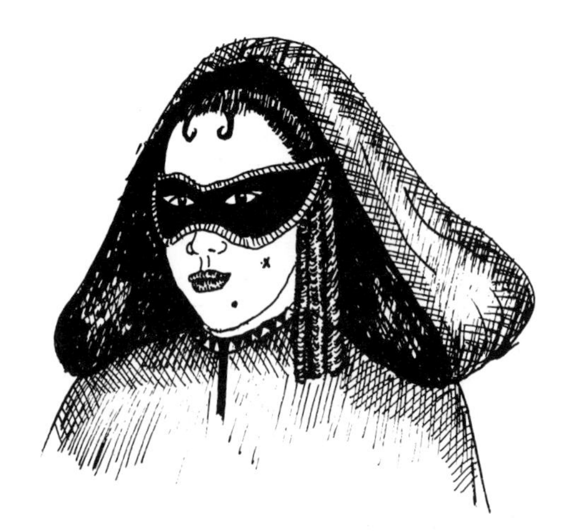

Fig. 4.37 Hooded cloak with half-mask adding a sense of mystery.

chivalry and gallantry, whereas puritan dress was plain and austere. Puritan beliefs forbade the use of lace, fine cloth and jewellery.

Dress

Fashion changed considerably during the Stuart reign, and whereas the Elizabethan period had been a time for ruffs and farthingales, this was now an era of lace and finery. Fashion became strongly influenced by French taste in 1625 when Charles I married Henrietta Maria of France, and later in 1660 during the restoration of Charles II from exile in France, fashions emulated the styles worn at the French court of Louis XIV.

Women

Women's fashions were less extravagant than men's, although they were just as elegant. The Elizabethan farthingale disappeared and was replaced by lace petticoats that gave a less artifical shape to the skirt, but the bodice was still tightly corseted to acquire the slender waist. The dresses were usually made from either satin or stiffened silk and it became fashionable to loop the ends of the skirt up to reveal the lace petticoats underneath (Fig. 4.36).

Women of fashion wore lace gloves and carried muffs, and fans. To add a touch of adventure into their lives when they went out they took to wearing half-masks under their large hooded cloaks (Fig. 4.37).

The Elizabethan ruff had been modified into a lace collar which bordered the low neck of the bodice. The sleeves of the dress were large and padded out, being the widest between the elbow and wrist. Shoes were similar to those worn in the Elizabethan period, except now they were likely to be adorned with fancy buckles.

Puritan dress consisted of black and white or dark plain garments with large white collars. The Puritans considered the frills and finery of women's clothes to be corrupt and evil.

Men

Cavalier dress was rich and flamboyant. The doublet disappeared and was replaced by loose trousers fastened to a short, waisted coat. The trousers were either tied at the knee with ribbons or were tucked inside large leather boots that reached to the thigh, called 'funnel boots'. The clothes were highly decorated with silk, lace and ribbons and the cavaliers usually wore a large lace collar attached to the neck of the coat (see Fig. 4.36).

Waistcoats became popular, being worn long like a coat at first. Then shorter versions became fashionable, and ties made an appearance worn round the neck loosely like a scarf. Later this developed into the 'cravat'. Cavaliers also carried swords, looking glasses and snuff boxes tucked away in their waistcoats.

Puritan dress was much plainer and totally practical in design, with absolutely no superfluous trimmings, apart from the large, white collar.

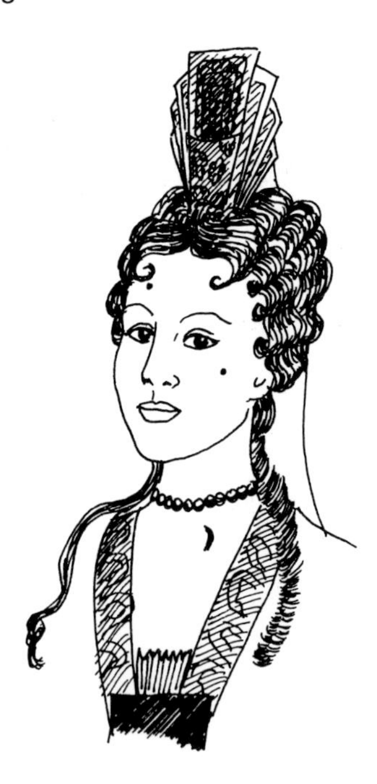

Fig. 4.38 'Fontange' or 'tower' headdress.

Hair styles and hats

Women

The majority of women did not wear hats, except occasionally a small black taffeta hood or a small lace bonnet when they went out. The favoured hair style of early Stuart fashion was that adopted by Charles I's French wife, Henrietta Maria. It was parted in the middle, flattened on top, then frizzed and curled each side of the head. Sometimes the hair at the crown or nape was coiled round into a bun. Ribbons were often used in the hair, and there was a fashion for love-locks, which were curls of hair worn at the temples, sides of the face or at the nape of the neck (see Fig. 4.37).

Later, towards the end of the 17th century a fashion was introduced from France of a headdress that grew to become very large. It was the 'fontange' or 'tower' headdress that started off as a small lace cap but developed into a tall, wired framework attached to the head and covered with silks and lace (Fig. 4.38).

Puritan women wore their hair shorter and neatly tucked away under a plain black, or dark coloured bonnet.

Men

The hair was worn long and curly (Fig. 4.39) and men took to wearing 'periwigs' in and outside the home. Sometimes the long curls were divided at

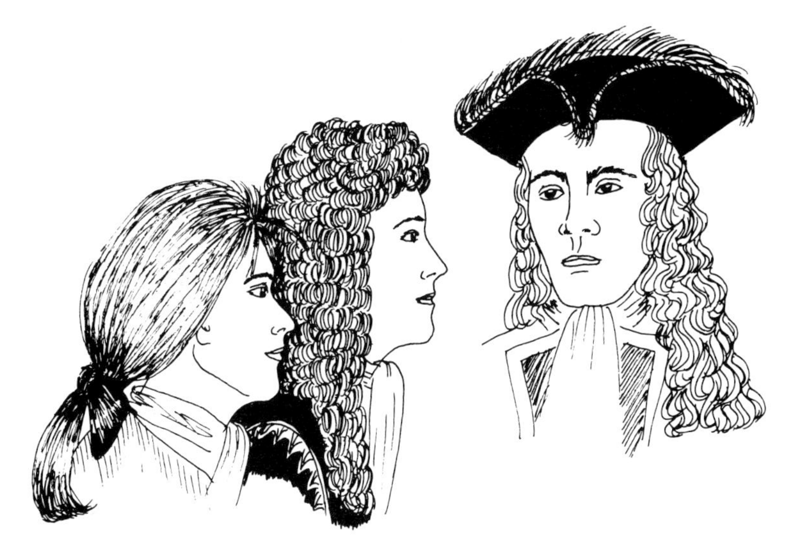

Fig. 4.39 Men's hair fashions – 'Tom Jones' pony-tail, 'periwig' and 'tricorne' hat.

the back and tied with ribbons or bows. Some men, in particular soldiers and travellers, began to tie back the flowing hair at the nape of the neck into a pony-tail like the one worn by the pop singer Tom Jones in the 1960s. The fashion for earrings still survived.

Hats were also very popular in and outside the home. The most popular was the 'tricorne' or 'cocked hat', which had three points to the rim.

Most fashionable men owned wigs of different types. Apart from the 'periwig', which was light, there was a 'full-bottomed' wig, which was a heavier, elaborate affair that must have been extremely restricting to wear. Towards the end of the century the wigs started to become double-peaked in the front and rose to quite a height. The hair was usually cropped quite short underneath so as to give the wigs a good fit, as well as to make the head cooler. Wigs were very expensive and it was common for small boys to be employed in snatching them off passing gentlemen in the street.

Beards went out of fashion, and a thin moustache, resembling that of Charles II, became popular.

Puritan men wore their hair cropped short, and wore the 'cocked hat' but without any feathers or trimmings.

Cosmetics and make-up

Women

Fashionable ladies wore quite heavy, elaborate make-up. White chalk was powdered onto the face, cheeks were rouged red and lips also reddened. It became fashionable for women to wear 'plumpers' which were made of cork and placed inside the mouth to fill out the cheeks, giving the face a plump appearance of youth.

It also became fashionable for ladies to shave off their eyebrows and replace them with mouse-skin, glued onto the forehead. Patches were still very popular and were now worn in a variety of shapes, (see Fig. 4.38) for example, moons, stars, or even in the shape of coach and horses.

Men

Although men wore extremely elaborate dress adorned with lace and ribbons, surprisingly the only make-up they wore was rouged cheeks.

4.9 18TH CENTURY – THE GEORGIAN PERIOD

The 18th century saw two distinct extremes in fashion and styles from the early part of the century to the later part. In the early 18th century the desire for elegance persisted from the 17th century, which was apparent in the paintings, dress, furniture and architecture of the period. The Baroque style of the late 17th century had displayed a desire to simulate the elegance of Classical art but instead resulted in stiff, formal representation. The Rococo style which developed in the early 18th century brought a much lighter, frivolous approach to fashion and seemed to concentrate solely on the surface decoration, to the extreme of becoming ostentatious. Portraits of this period can been seen by looking at the work of artists Watteau and Boucher.

The French Revolution in 1789 cut off the French dominance over fashion styles, and for a while English fashion looked to the countryside for inspiration. This produced a very simple, natural countrified style. This look was made possible by the invention of machines that could make light fabrics in large quantities from the cotton imported from the colonies.

Towards the end of the century the fascination for Classical Antiquity developed into the neo-classical or Regency period, and fashion took on a totally simplistic tack, harking back to the simple, symmetrical styles of the ancient Greeks.

Dress

Women

Early 18th century dress hardly changed from the fashions of the late 17th century. If anything it grew to extremes, with the dome-shaped hoops and panniers spreading extremely wide (Fig. 4.40), causing chaos in restricted areas such as doorways, pathways and corridors. The 'manteau' was the formal gown that was worn over these large panniers, and was made from heavy brocaded materials. This was later replaced by lighter, softer materials, such as silks, satins and indeed cotton, which had become popular after being introduced from the colonies. The neckline usually consisted of a deep,

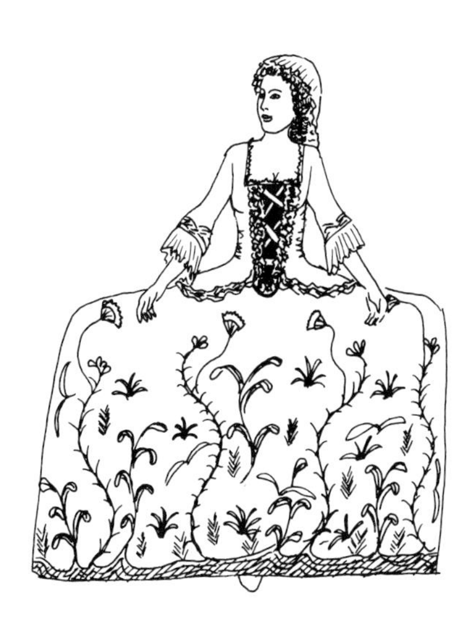

Fig. 4.40 'Manteau' gown worn over panniers.

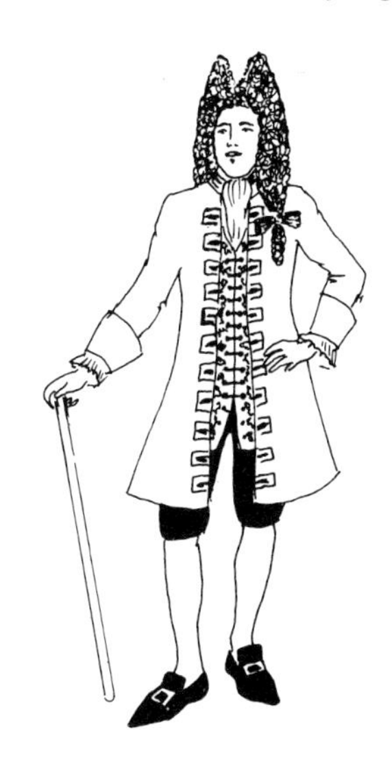

Fig. 4.41 Early 18th century men's dress.

square décolletage, and it became very popular to wear tucked inside concealed pockets fragrant herbs and perfume sachets, or 'nose-gays', which were bunches of fresh flowers kept in small bottles of water nestled between the bosoms. Corsets were still worn and were usually stiffened with whalebone.

Fashion changed slightly around the mid-1750s when the large hoops and panniers were replaced by smaller hoops or a type of small bustle that padded out the bottom. This decrease in framework underneath the skirts made them reach lower onto the floor, causing a train to flow behind.

Fashion dolls were sent from country to country (usually coming from France) clothed in the latest fashions and hair styles so that the fashion-conscious and wealthy could keep up to the minute with the latest styles.

Later, about 1790, fashion totally changed. Corsets, whalebone and layers of fine satins were discarded and replaced by the barest layer of fine linen, light cottons and silks. The neo-classical fashions were based on a 'chemise' cut in the style of ancient Greek dress. This was a high-waisted flimsy tunic draped over the body in the simplest way, with only the support of an elasticated band worn under the lower part of the bosom to give the required décolletage (Fig. 4.42). It was the least amount of clothes women had adorned in this climate since perhaps the ancient Roman Britons.

Woollen shawls would be worn over the dresses, and flat leather sandals criss-crossing around the ankle.

Men

Early 18th century dress did not change dramatically. Men wore brocaded silks, long buttoned waistcoats stiffened with buckram, and double-breasted

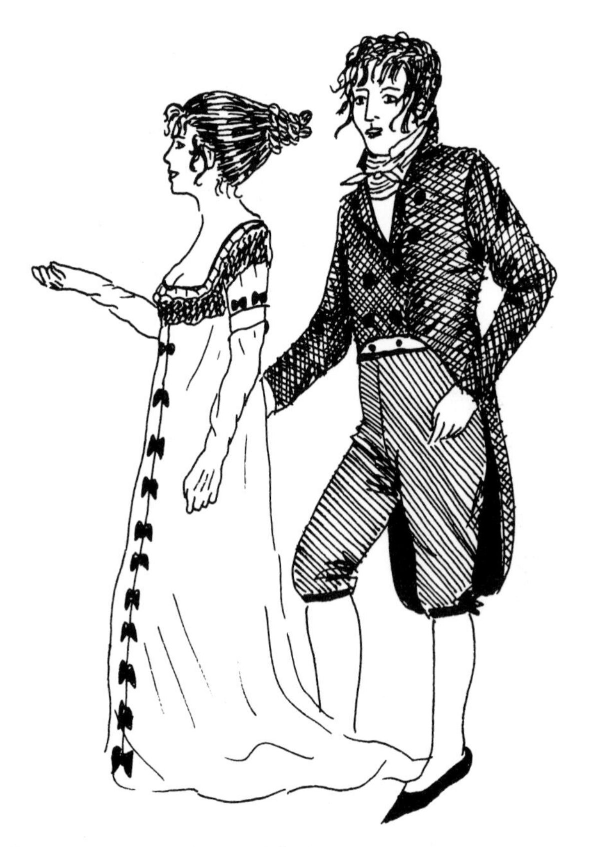

Fig. 4.42 Neo-classical fashions in the late 18th century.

coats (see Fig. 4.41). The neo-classical styles only changed women's fashions although men's fashions did take on a more simple, countrified look. They adapted the Englishman's hunting coat, with exaggerated tails at the back. They wore looser-fitting breeches and knee-length boots. Waistcoats became shorter and the height of the collar rose. Neck-cloths or ties became exaggerated and took on the appearance of a protruding bib. The stiff, formal figure gave way to more of a natural, dishevelled appearance (see Fig. 4.42).

Hair styles

Women

During the early 1700s, after the death of Queen Anne, the 'fontange' and 'tour' headdresses disappeared and hair styles became simple for a while. The hair was taken back off the face into a curled bun at the back of the head with one or two locks hanging below or laying over the shoulders. Small,

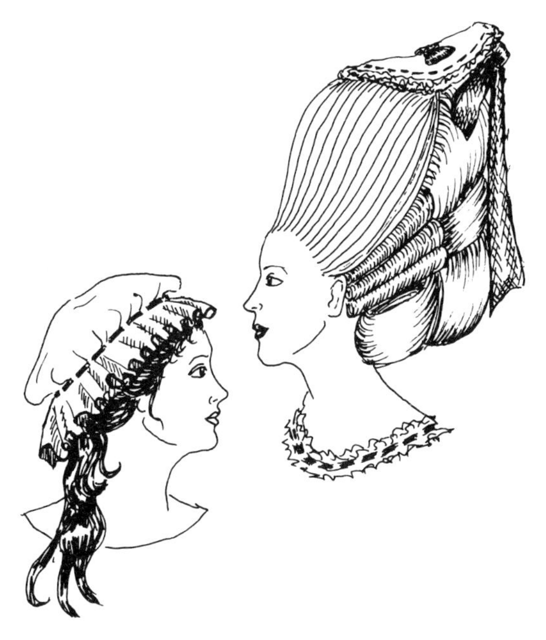

Fig. 4.43 Contrast of 18th century hair styles – early 'mob-caps' and the powdered wigs of the late 18th century.

round caps called 'pinners' became popular, then later 'mob-caps', which had tied strings under the chin called 'kissing strings' (Fig. 4.43).

Later, the French influence on fashion popularised the wearing of false hair and wigs, but only for the wealthy. Hairdressers or friseurs were in great demand by the aristocracy and were fearfully guarded. Coiffure was a serious business and took a painfully long time to complete. It was particularly popular to powder the hair white with wheatmeal flour, which was applied by spraying with hand bellows high above the head so that the flour would fall evenly over the hair. Rolls of horsehair, wool pads and wire supports were used to achieve particular hair styles (see Fig. 4.43).

The shapes and fashions of the hair styles at this time literally rose to ridiculous heights. Women would comb up their hair, both natural and false, to cover a horsehair pad that would be worn on the crown and then finish it off with rows of curls at the back. These curls were usually false, being curled into shape with heated clay rollers called 'bigoudis'. The entire arrangement was kept in place with pins and pomade (a gel-like substance that acted as a sort of glue and gave a good adhesion to the flour). The finished coiffure would then be decorated with ribbon, feathers, flowers. Some extreme styles would actually reach two or three feet in height and display such scenes as 'ducks on a lake', 'gardens of flowers', 'hunting scenes', or a 'seascape incorporating a galleon'. These hair designs proved problematic when the owners tried to move around. Ladies had to resort to hanging their heads out of carriages or even kneeling down in them in order not to disarray their artistic creations.

These coiffures were attended to by hairdressers, in the case of the wealthy about once a week, but for the less wealthy probably about once a month or worse. This caused hygiene problems. The pomatum that was used was based on beef marrow and often went rancid, attracting swarms of bugs and even nests of mice. Long head scratchers became widely used by both men and women.

Men

The chief characteristic of early 18th century dress for men was the wig (see Fig. 4.41). Wigs generally fell into two categories: those with 'queues' (hair hanging down the back) or those without. The most popular was the 'full-bottomed' wig, but the 'long-bob' and the 'short-bob' were also popular. These wigs were usually set in curls, powdered, and were extremely expensive. They became a vehicle to display wealth and were cherished to the extent of becoming a bequeathed item in a will. Wig-snatching became a common crime. Young boys hidden in carried baskets snatched a wig off a victim's head and beat a hasty retreat, selling it later for a profitable sum.

The wigs were sometimes worn tied at the back in a pig-tail and because of their length and volume were quite heavy to wear. It became more comfortable to wear the natural hair quite short or even to shave the hair completely, a device the ancient Egyptians also adopted for comfort.

Later, when the fashion changed to a more natural style the powdered wigs disappeared and were replaced by the hair being cut quite short and dressed forward (after the style adopted by Napoleon). This style was called the 'Brutus cut' and was intentionally dishevelled to give a windswept appearance. Side-burns also became popular (see Fig. 4.42).

Cosmetics and make-up

Make-up was used more by both sexes up until the latter half of the century. Faces were powdered white, in keeping with the whitened hair and to give a very stark look. Dark eyebrows were drawn over existing ones and lips were painted very red. The overall effect conjures up the theatrical picture of the ugly sisters in Cinderella (Fig. 4.44). Black or coloured patches were still popular in varying shapes: squares, hearts, diamonds etc., and were a successful way of drawing attention to a particular feature and the popularity of wearing cork 'plumpers' from the late 17th century continued. Men revived the Elizabethan fashion of wearing earrings.

4.10 19TH CENTURY

The 19th century saw a contrast of fashions, some to opposite extremes. The flimsy neo-classical female attire that was fashionable at the start of the century changed within thirty years to fashions that compelled women to

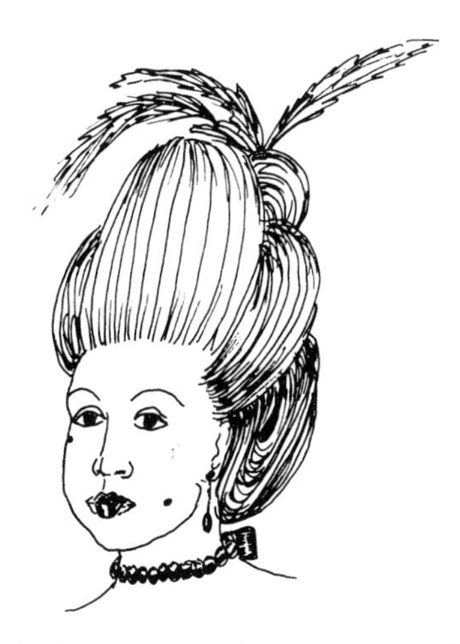

Fig. 4.44 18th century fashions in make-up – note the 'plumpers' worn in the cheeks to give a plump youthful appearance.

wear more clothes than they had ever before worn. In a way this reflected the times. The social and economic change activated by the Industrial Revolution gave rise to the budding 'middle class' in the 19th century. With their new found wealth they acquired a lifestyle that simulated the pleasures and fineries which had been a privilege of the aristocracy. Subsequently fads and fashions became available to more people. The century also saw advances in technology, which enabled the production of new and cheaper clothing materials.

An important invention which influenced fashion in the later part of the 19th century was that of the sewing machine. Until then gowns had been hand-stitched and extremely expensive. Now, with the sewing machine, mass-production of clothing became easier and therefore cheaper, reaching a wider range of customer.

Dress

Women

The neo-classical style of dress that became popular in the latter part of the 18th century continued into the early part of the 19th century with slight modifications. Napoleon's expedition to Egypt generated an influence of orientialism in fashions, which was blended with a strong Spanish influence.

Styles changed about 1822, when the waist returned and inevitably so did the corset. The smallness of the waist was emphasised by the fullness of the skirt and the puffiness of the shoulders, which resembled the Tudor style of dress. The skirt grew fuller by the 1850s, so much so that it demanded the support of the caged crinoline (which again resembled a past fashion; that of the Elizabethan 'farthingale') and the vast hooped expanse of skirt gave an

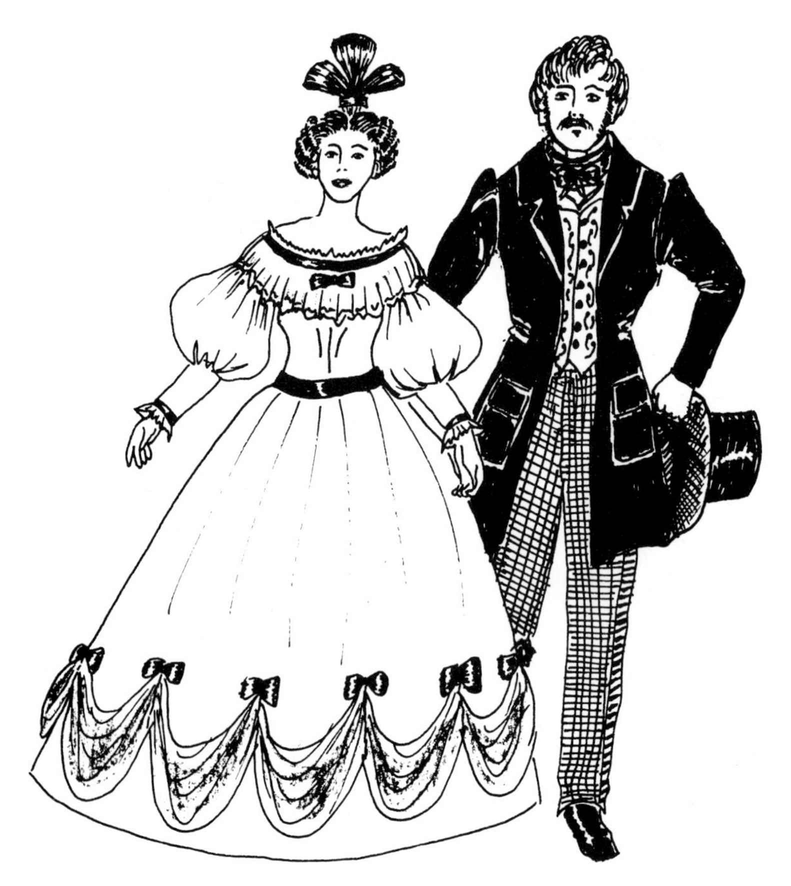

Fig. 4.45 Early 19th century fashions – crinoline and 'Apollo knot' and male fashions.

impression of gliding to the petite female frame underneath as the woman walked (Fig. 4.45). The crinoline grew to its largest size by the 1860s.

The style changed around 1870. The large crinoline became flattened in the front and moved its expanse of material round to the back. This was the beginning of the 'bustle', although it did not become very popular until later when a modified version of a more horizontal 'bustle' became fashionable in the 1880s (Fig. 4.46). The 'bustle' required a much smaller wire frame attached around the waist with a two-or three-tiered wire support at the small of the back. When the skirt was laid over this it emphasised and flattered the curve of the back and the female shape.

At this time the French influence on fashion, lost during the French Revolution, revived, especially since the popular English-born designer Charles Worth lived and worked in Paris. He totally dominated *haute couture*. Newly invented aniline dyes allowed brighter colours in fabrics, and blues, mauves and pinks were fashionable until the death of Prince Albert

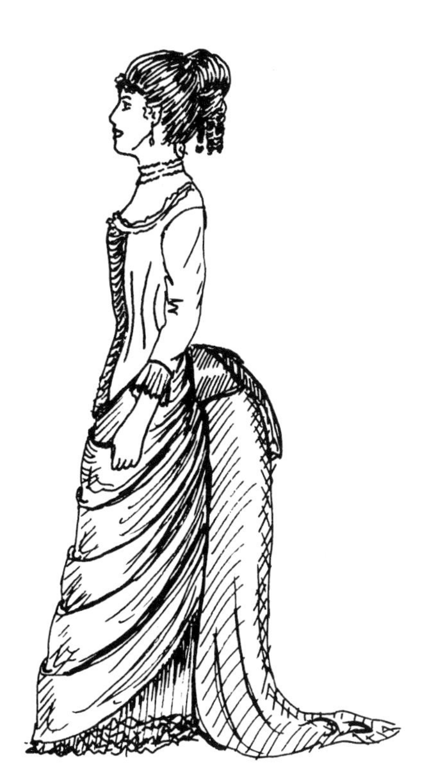

Fig. 4.46 'Bustle'.

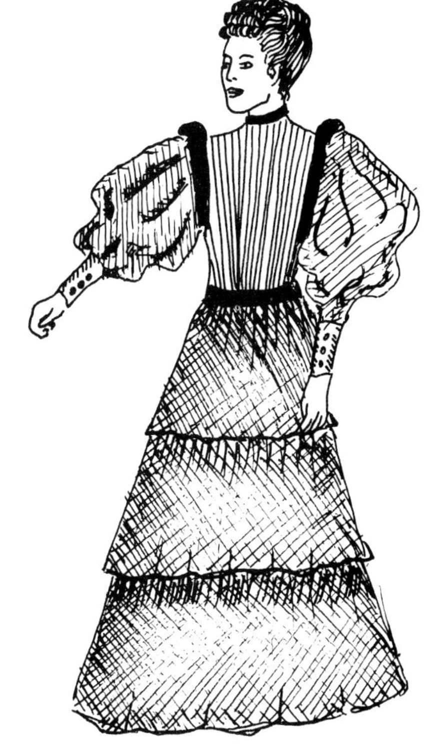

Fig. 4.47 'Leg-of-mutton' sleeves.

when Queen Victoria adopted black as a token of respect and was imitated by her loyal subjects.

Women became very fond of sport, such as tennis, and particularly cycling. A new kind of fashion emerged through this hobby, that of practicality. In 1862, women for the first time wore a form of 'bloomer' that had first been introduced earlier in the century by an American, Amelia Bloomer. These had been rejected then, but were now adopted as they allowed easier movement of the legs.

The 'bustle' disappeared by 1895, and the skirt style returned to a smoother cone shape that had been popular earlier in the century. The focus, was once again on the sleeves. Huge, billowing 'leg-of-mutton' sleeves became the fashion (Fig. 4.47).

Men

Unlike the female fashions, men's fashions were dominated by a strong English influence. This originated from a notorious male character who lived in the early 19th century, Beau Brummel. He epitomised the so-called 'dandy', whose total existence was concerned with appearance and perfection in detail (see Fig. 4.45). He set high standards and from London's Savile Row emerged master craftsmen in tailoring. He also was responsible for the popularity of mixing colours together, for instance, he would wear a yellow waistcoat with a green jacket. High collars and cravats were fashionable, as well as tight fitting pants and knee-high boots. Clothes were an indication of wealth and hats were worn by most men and acted as a status symbol. A top hat called a 'bicorne' was worn by the upper- and middle-class men, although some of the middle classes would prefer to wear a 'tam-o-shanter' cap with a leather peak. The working class wore bowlers or 'billy-cocks (similar to the city gent's well-known bowler). The poorer man would make a hat to cover his head and only the very poor would go bare-headed. Most men carried either a cane or an umbrella.

The Romantic movement and the Pre-Raphaelites

Another movement that was going on simultaneously was the Romantic movement that had started in the 18th century. The Romantics, inspired by poets such as Lord Byron, Tennyson and Keats, rejected bourgeois values and sought spiritual fulfillment and a simple life-style. Their beliefs were similar to those of the neo-classical movement at the end of the 18th century which had revived the values of the ancient civilisations and also to those of the Pre-Raphaelite Brotherhood. The Pre-Raphaelites were a group of artists and writers, amongst whom was Rossetti, who believed that art had become contrived, artificial and pompous. They sought for the purity and truth they associated with the great medieval painters who had lived before the artist Raphael revolutionised painting styles during the Renaissance. A famous designer associated with this movement was William Morris, who recaptured some of the medieval decorative arts in many of his designs.

The male fashions of this movement were loose, plain clothes that paid no attention to finery or decoration. Darker, mystical colours were favoured: mauves, browns, blacks, which played off against the favoured pallor of complexion to create a haunted look. The men did not wear hats, and the hair had a very unkempt appearance. The female fashions rejected the tight corsetry and disfigurement of contemporary fashions and sought the simplicity of loose-fitting garments like those worn in medieval times, without any decoration or trimming (Fig. 4.48). Their hair was left natural as were their complexions, although some did resort to drastic measures by drinking vinegar to acquire the desirable pallor.

Hair styles

Women

The hair styles at the beginning of the century flattered the neo-classical clothes. The hair would be simply dressed high into a coil or bandeau, or sometimes it was cut short and worn in curls bedecked with pearls or decorative combs. White wigs also became fashionable. During the period of oriental influence on fashions women wore turbans with ostrich feathers and

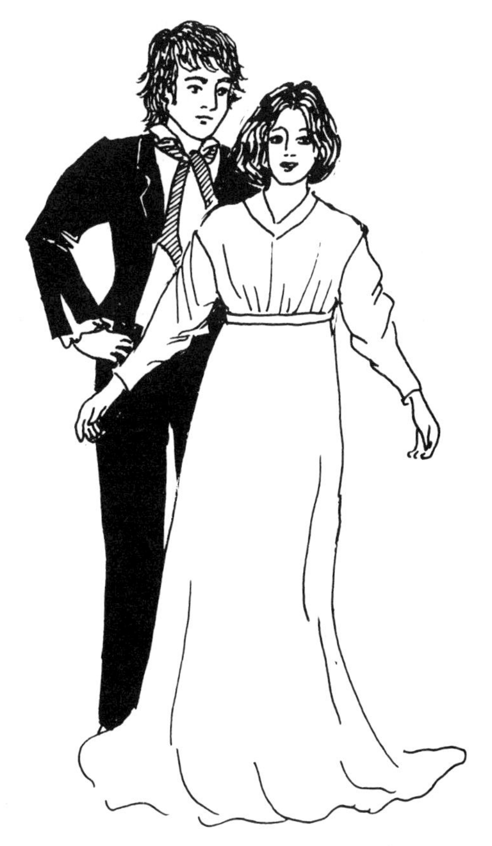

Fig. 4.48 The fashions of the Romantic movement.

pearls. Hats were worn earlier in the century but they were quite small and bonnet-shaped. Later, with the rise of the crinoline more elaborate hair styles emerged. Curls, ringlets and 'apollo knots' requiring ample use of false hair were adorned with bows and feathers (see Fig. 4.45). Black hair was very fashionable and an abundance was imported from France and Italy. The fashion changed within twenty years. Blonde hair became the vogue, so again ample false hair was imported, now from Northern France and Germany.

The Victorian bun or top-knot became popular. This required large amounts of hair, that was loosely drawn up to a bun or knot at the crown, and its main aim was to give the appearance of fullness and smoothness. Most Victorian hair styles had certain details in common. Most had centre partings, and perhaps one of the most characteristic styles of the Victorian era was the 'chignon', where the hair was parted in the middle, drawn over the ears and arranged into a bun at the nape of the neck (Fig. 4.49). With the emphasis at the back of the head the 'cache peigne' became popular. This consisted of looped ribbons fixed to a stiff piece of net. It was attached to the plaits or bun originally as an attempt to conceal the joins in the plaids or the combs, but it gained popularity.

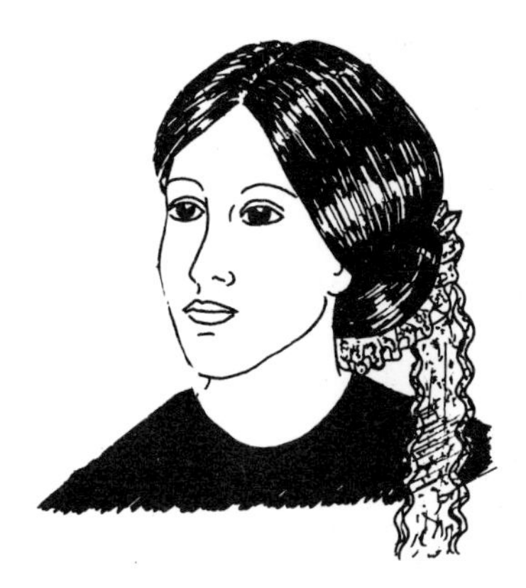

Fig. 4.49 'Chignon' worn with 'cache peigne' headdress.

An important development in hairdressing took place in 1870 when a French hairdresser, Marcel Grateau, perfected a technique with the help of heated irons to produce a natural-looking wave that was named after him, the 'Marcel' wave.

Caps and headdresses were extremely popular in the Victorian period, and the 'snood' of the 13th and 14th centuries reappeared, encasing the 'chignons' in hanging nets. The popularity of straw grew, and straw hats or boaters became very popular.

Men

Earlier in the century older men and professionals still wore short, 'queued' wigs, although they were constantly losing popularity due to the tax on hair powders that was introduced in 1795. Younger men sported the dishevelled 'Brutus crop'. Later, the hair was worn longer and curled in a neater style that was usually parted in the centre and kept tame by the use of macassar oil. The introduction of the fashionable high collar required the hair at the back to be cut shorter. Most men were clean-shaven with heavy side-whiskers, although it became very fashionable later on for men to wear a moustache. Special moustache waxes consisting of a mixture of beeswax and pomade were used.

Cosmetics and make-up

Earlier in the century cosmetics and make-up were a little more popular than later on. Men blanched the backs of their hands to give a whitened appearance, and rouged their cheeks by using either walnut juice or rouge. Rouged cheeks became less popular for women on the other hand, as the favoured complexion was languid and pale. A colourful face was considered by Victorian values to be vulgar and a sign of prostitution.

4.11 20TH CENTURY

The 20th century has been a time of great change, greater than in any previous century. The First World War (1914–1918) and the Second World War (1939–1945) brought about immense economic and social restructuring both in Britain and overseas. Industrial strength, together with the creation of the Welfare State and compulsory education for all have helped to improve the standard of life for ordinary people. Women have acquired improved economic status and the vote. Advances in medicine have helped to lengthen our life-span, communication and travel have broadened our cultural understanding, and science has heightened our awareness and understanding of our existence on our planet.

The invention of the mass media and the ability to manufacture clothing cheaply have made the world of fashion accessible to everyone. This, in turn, has stimulated faster change and a greater variety of fashions than ever before.

1900–1910–The Edwardian period

Women

King Edward VII was very fashion-conscious and set the pace for men's fashions in this period. His influence also dominated female fashions as he particularly favoured the shape of the 'mature woman'. This involved women wearing an artificial, distorted corset that thrust the bust forward, tightened the waist and pushed the hips backward resulting in an S-shape (Fig. 4.50), which must have been agony to wear and did dreadful damage to the internal organs. It is no wonder that a characteristic image of the Edwardian lady was that she constantly fainted.

Women had a passion for lace to decorate their dresses, but for those who could not afford the lace Irish crochet was a good substitute. The popular colours reflected a new age. The sombre, dark colours of late Victorian dress gave way to pastel shades of pink, blues, greens and mauves.

The S-shape softened slightly in 1908 when a modification to the corset set a new shape of straighter hips. The 'Empire' gown became the fashion, and with it wide-rimmed hats were worn to make the hips look even slimmer.

Another characteristic of Edwardian dress was the high collar that extended to under the chin and was complemented by hair styles that were swept up off the neck and dressed on top of the head. The front hair was usually worn high, dressed over crepe pads, and this was called the 'pompadour' style (Fig. 4.51).

Men

Men's fashions followed the preferences of the King. The city gent style was favoured. This included a high collar with bow tie, waistcoat, straight jacket

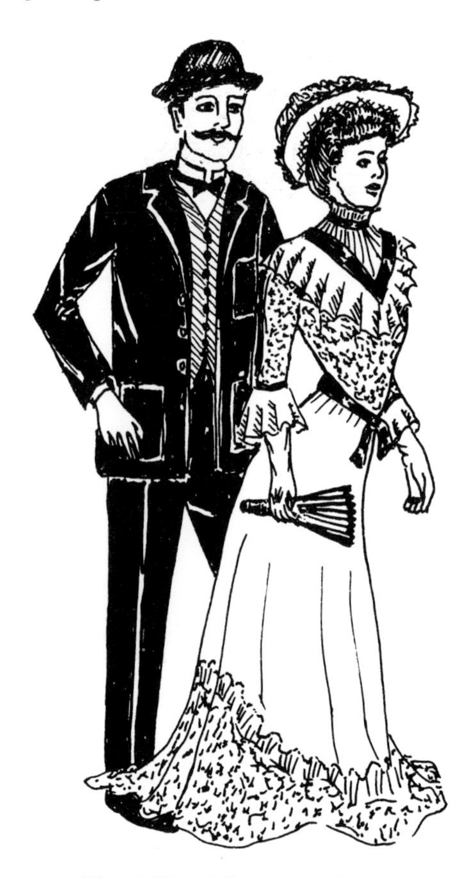

Fig. 4.50 Edwardian fashions.

with unpadded shoulders and straight sleeves, and narrow trouser legs with turn-ups. Men's hair was worn short above the collar, and usually parted in the middle or at the side, and oiled. The popularity for side whiskers had disappeared, but most men wore moustaches (see Fig. 4.50).

1910–1920

In 1910 a revolution in fashion began. An adventurous French fashion designer, Paul Poiret, had become inspired by the 1908 Russian ballet performance in Paris of Scheherezade, directed by Diaghilev, with superb oriental costumes designed by Leon Bakst. Poiret was entranced and from his imagination came a totally new shape for women. The theme was oriental, and the colours were garish reds, oranges, lemons and brilliant blues. 'Colour is liberation' Matisse had announced, disclosing the philosophy behind the Fauvist movement in painting, and Poiret was declared the 'Fauve of fashion'. The shape of Poiret's new woman was like an up-turned triangle. Wide, loose fabrics swathed the body and narrowed towards the ankles (Fig. 4.52). The

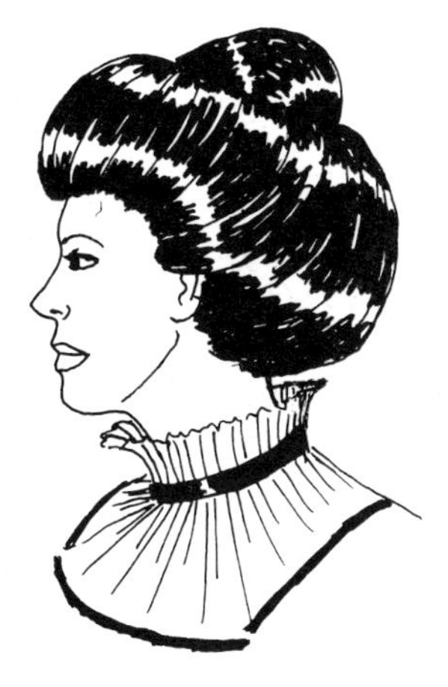

Fig. 4.51 Characteristic Edwardian 'pompadour' hair style.

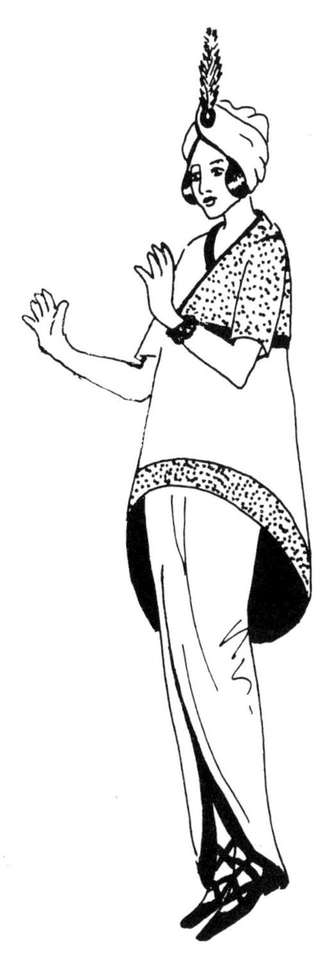

Fig. 4.52 Poiret's oriental style with the 'hobble' skirt.

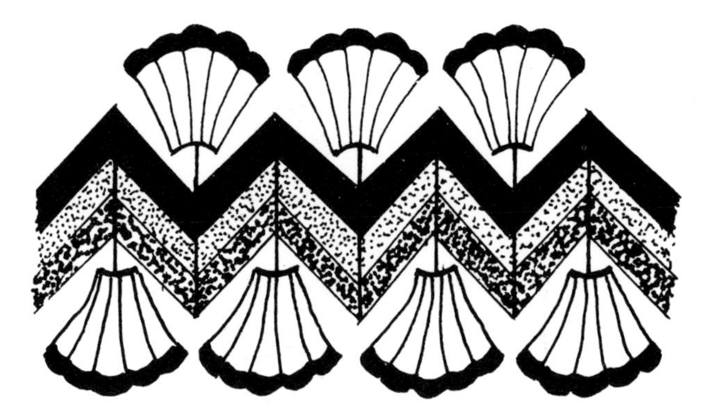

Fig. 4.53 Example of Art Deco design.

tight restricting corsetry was no longer necessary and was abandoned, to be replaced by the new lighter rubber girdles that he had also devised. The new 'hobble-skirts' had liberated the body but at the same time had now restricted the feet. (This was later modified by slitting the skirts in the front or at the sides to allow more freedom of movement.) High waists, straighter skirts, tunic overdresses, turbans, kimonos: all these new styles created a new, younger, thinner shape, offset by new oriental fashions in headwear and accessories, silk turbans, scarves, feathers, etc.

The First World War, 1914–1918, brought everything including the fashion world to a standstill. It did not pick up again until about 1919, when fashion designers realised that women, after the rationing during the war, and with their increased interest in sport, were in better shape. The hourglass figure that had once seemed so desirable now looked comical. Fashion suddenly focused on the younger woman instead of the middle-aged woman.

1920–1930

Women

When fashion did pick up after the war it reflected the mood of the times. The desire to escape from the depression of the war years spurred fashion designers such as Poiret, Coco Chanel and Shiapirelli to launch the new mood of the emancipated woman.

The styles dictated a straighter, shorter silhouette, which seemed to simulate boyish charm. The new 'androgynous look' of the emancipated woman had arrived.

The clothes hung on the body, hiding any suggestions of a female figure underneath and resembling a tubular framework, and, as if suddenly all social rules had gone out of the window, hemlines started to climb up the leg. For the first time women began to show their ankles. Then as the decade went on the hemlines went higher until about 1925–26 when they were up to the knee. There was a public outcry and religious condemnation, but to no

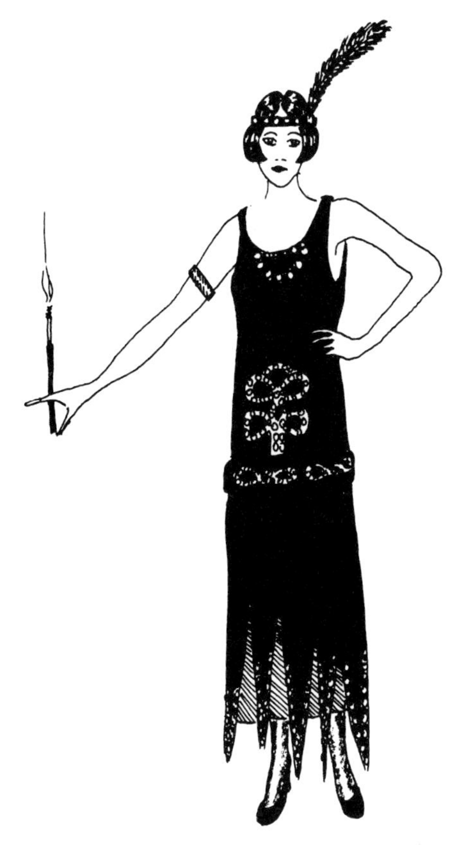

Fig. 4.54 The 'flapper' look of the 1920s.

avail; these were women with a mission. Not only did the length of the dress shock, women also started to smoke, wear provocative make-up and do the Charleston dance.

In 1923 Lord Carnarvon discovered the tomb of Tutankhamen in Egypt. This inspired a new design movement, Art Deco, which influenced fashions, furniture and the decorative arts with simplicity of line, geometric and angular shapes (Fig. 4.53). The new 'flapper' look was completed with a long string of pearls, feather boa, cigarette holder, and head band (Fig. 4.54).

The new emancipated woman was completed when the long, feminine tresses were shorn to shorter, boyish hair styles, such as the short 'French bob', and the more dramatic 'shingle' and 'Eton crop' (Figs 4.55 and 4.56). Most fashionable women would go to barber shops to have their hair cut, sometimes even shorter than the men themselves. The short hair styles seemed to be the subject of many domestic rows and many married women would compromise by cutting the front hair short, but leaving the hair at the back long so it could be wound up into a bun or a coil (Fig. 4.57). Fringes were extremely popular.

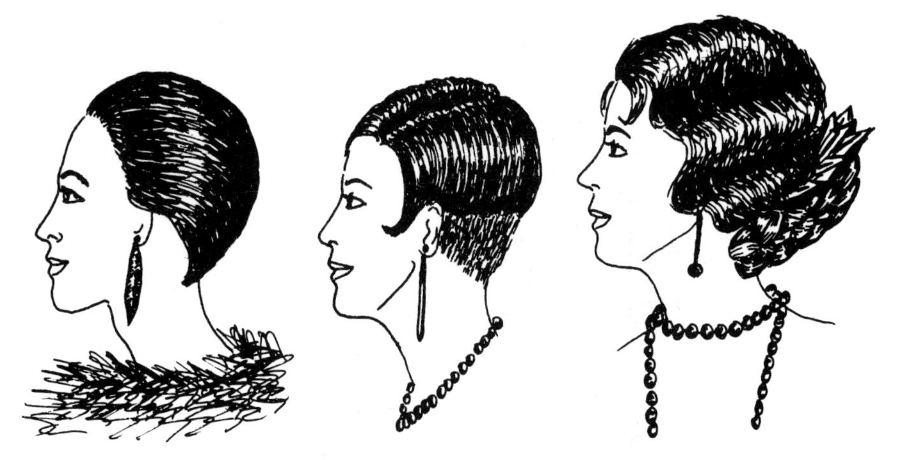

Fig. 4.55 'Eton crop'. **Fig. 4.56** 'Shingle' cut. **Fig. 4.57** Compromise style.

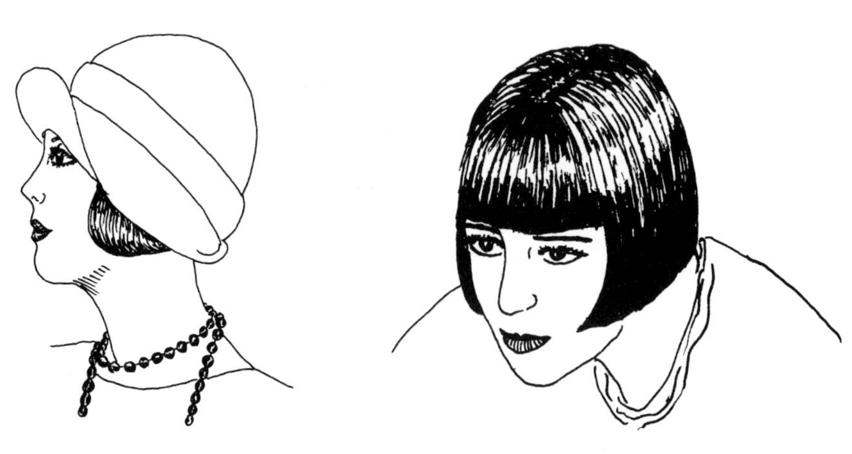

Fig. 4.58 'Cloche' hat. **Fig. 4.59** The 'Clara Bow' look.

Hats lost their elegance, size and popularity, except for the 'cloche' hat, which was an important part of the twenties' look (Fig. 4.58).

Another important influence on fashion in the 1920s was the first glimpse of glamour through the silent films of Hollywood. The dark, Egyptian looks of Clara Bow became the desirable image, with black kohl eyes and Cupid bow lips (Fig. 4.59). Later, towards 1929, women's fashions started to soften slightly. The line was not so harsh and the hemlines dropped to mid-calf.

Men

Fashions for men also changed after the war years. The waistcoat lost favour and was replaced by the double-breasted jacket. But one of the most outrageous changes, in line with the extremities of female dress, was the

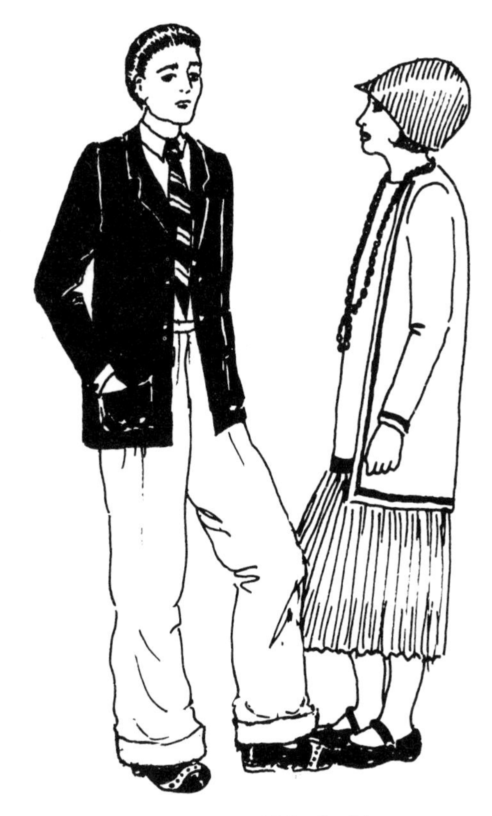

Fig. 4.60 1920s fashions.

onset of 'Oxford bags' – huge, baggy trousers which often covered the shoe. 'Plus fours', baggy knee-length bloomers, were also popular (Fig. 4.60).

Flat caps became popular, and men's hair was worn short and combed straight back (Fig. 4.61). Most men were clean shaven. The Prince of Wales set the fashion, favouring wide lapels and padded shoulders with a tighter-fitting jacket and wide trousers.

1930–1940

Women

The early 1930s saw a softer, more feminine female shape in fashions. Although the silhouette still had a tubular shape, the styles gave an indication of the curve of the waist, and the skirts had begun to be cut on the bias so that the garments clung to the hips. The hemline had dropped, and the focus now had moved to the new backless dress (Fig. 4.62). Black, navy and cream were still favourite colours, but also popular were duck egg blue, peach and shocking pink. Large wrap-over coats were also fashionable. There was still a

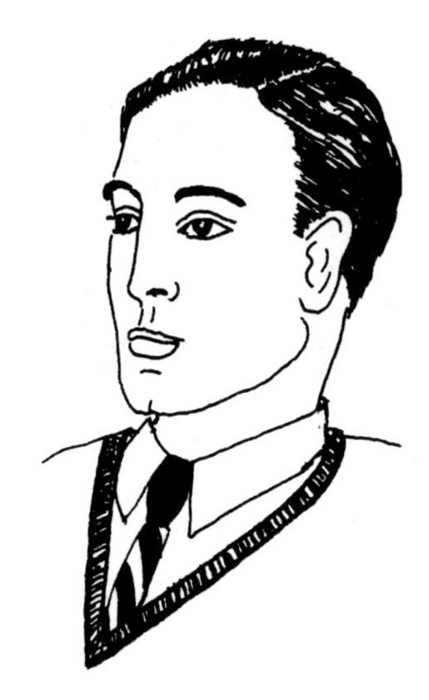

Fig. 4.61 Male look of the 1920s.

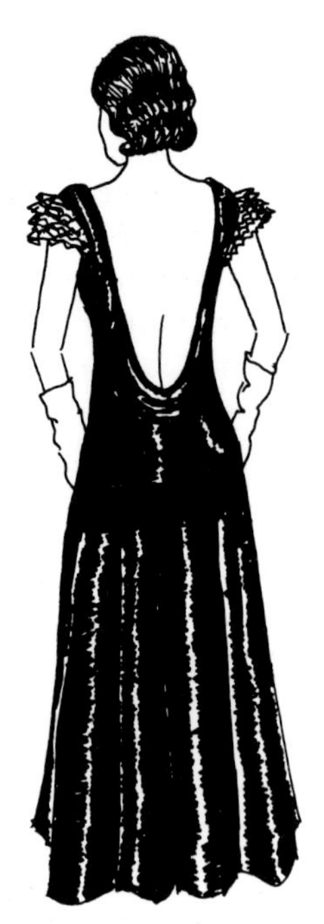

Fig. 4.62 The backless dress of the 1930s.

trend for masculine clothes, perhaps best illustrated by the man's suit worn by Marlene Dietrich, which epitomised the emancipated woman.

The shape shifted slightly in the mid-1930s from the tube to the pyramid. Wide shoulders and slender hips became fashionable, and so did the tall,

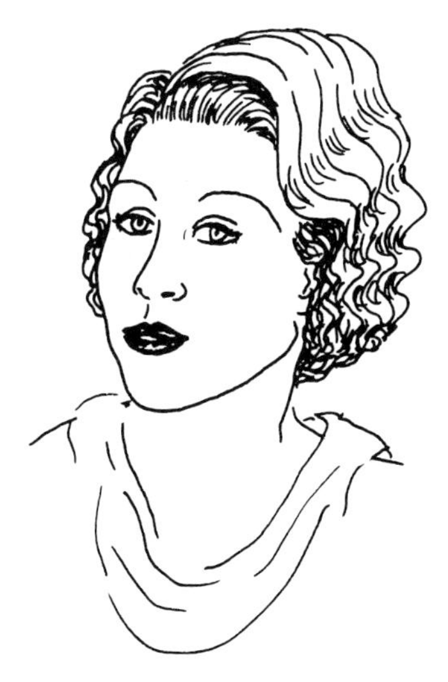

Fig. 4.63 The 1930s look.

slender shape. This was often enhanced by a hair style worn close to the head, with a small hat cocked to one side. Permanent waving had become popular and many styles had 'end perming', where the front hair was kept short and the back was longer with just the ends curled (Fig. 4.63). The mid-30s saw an influx of small, sometimes strange shaped hats as well as accessories inspired by the Surrealist movement in painting.

Another interesting shift was that fashion trends were now set by the images of Hollywood film stars rather than pure fashion garments. Women wanted the 'look', and with the added bonus of ready-to-wear clothes that were fast becoming available, they found they could achieve it. Greta Garbo, Marlene Dietrich, Joan Crawford and Jean Harlow look-a-likes emerged. Pencil-thin eyebrows framed heavy lidded, half-asleep looks, or outlined eyes and rich, luscious lips strived to find some identity. Blonde hair became very fashionable, and many women dyed their own hair, with harsh bleaches.

Men

Fashions had steadily become more informal and men too enjoyed the influence of Hollywood. Slick good looks, a pencil moustache and short, neat hair seemed to echo the American gangster image, but generally most men still wore wide trousers, and knitted sleeveless jumpers became fashionable, worn over a shirt and tie. 'Zoot suits' became a trend amongst the younger men and were influenced by bygone jazz days. Wide lapels, double-breasted, three-quarter length jackets, narrower trousers were worn with jazzy coloured ties, and a trilby hat.

The Second World War (1939–1945) brought the world of fashion to a grinding halt as all resources were poured into the war effort.

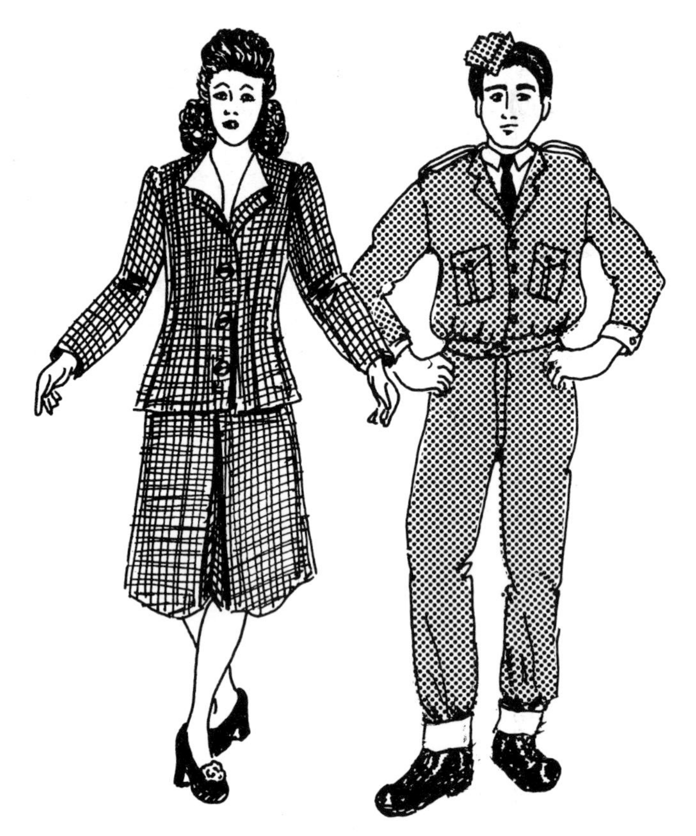

Fig. 4.64 'Utility' clothing and forces uniform of the 1940s.

1940–1950

Fashions during the Second World War did not change very much. The basic silhouette stayed plain and square, which was an inevitable influence of the uniforms. Colours were also plain (green, blue and khaki) because of the lack of dyes. Cloth and buttons were restricted per garment. This range of fashions was labelled 'Utility' clothing, and these were the only clothes available for the exchange of rationing coupons (Fig. 4.64).

Women who went to work in factories for the war effort wore turbans and snoods for safety. These replaced the fancy small hats, and dungarees and trousers replaced the delicate dresses. Practicality suddenly became more important (Fig. 4.65).

The lack of fashion interest meant that more attention was paid to the hair in these war years. Most women grew their hair longer and the long page-boy favoured by Hollywood star Veronica Lake was popular (Fig. 4.66).

After the war rationing and austerity prevailed. It was not until 1947 that a new mood emerged, epitomised by a French designer, Christian Dior, in his 'New Look' (Fig. 4.67). It was a nostalgic harking back to securer times and

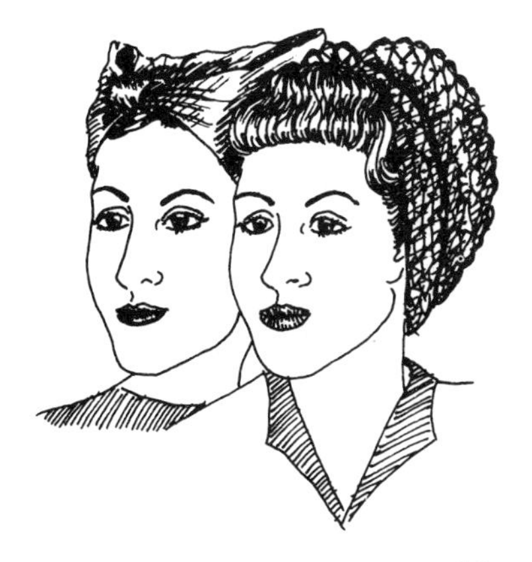

Fig. 4.65 Practicality in headdress for factory work – the turban and snood.

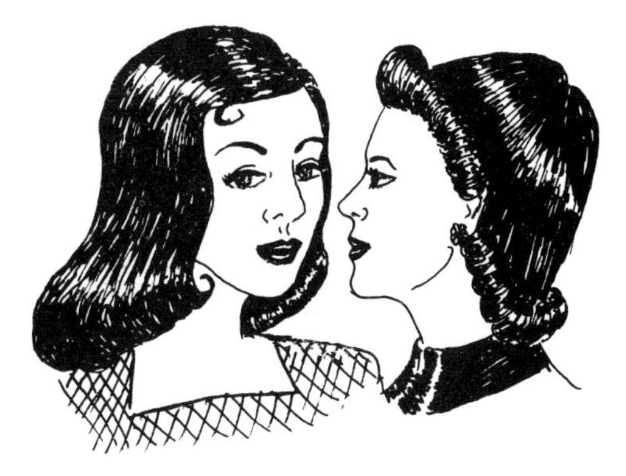

Fig. 4.66 Popular hair styles during the 1940s.

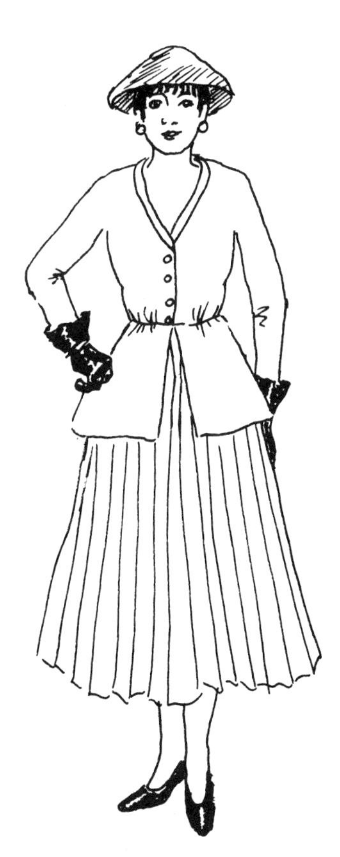

Fig. 4.67 Christian Dior's new look launched in 1947.

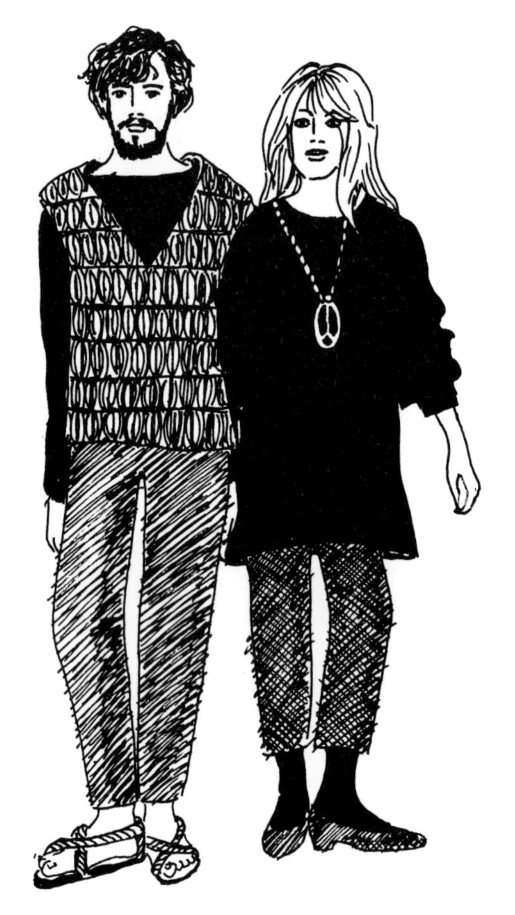

Fig. 4.68 Beatniks.

was just what the war-weary public needed. The wasp waist returned with the help of waist corsets (waspies), along with full skirts, a softer shoulder line and a new emphasis on the bust. The female figure had returned.

The new image also revitalised interest in hair styles, and shorter styles became popular, in particular the 'urchin' cut, shaggy and shingled. Ponytails became popular for the younger females as a direct influence from America, also bleached streaks became the rage. An interest in hats returned. Small hats with nets were worn perched on one side and berets were popular.

Men after the war were issued with 'demob' suits and were glad to be in civilian clothes after years of uniforms.

1950–1960

After Dior's new look an array of different styles swamped the fashion world, focusing attention on either the waist, knees, hips or hemline. Most of them were very short-lived.

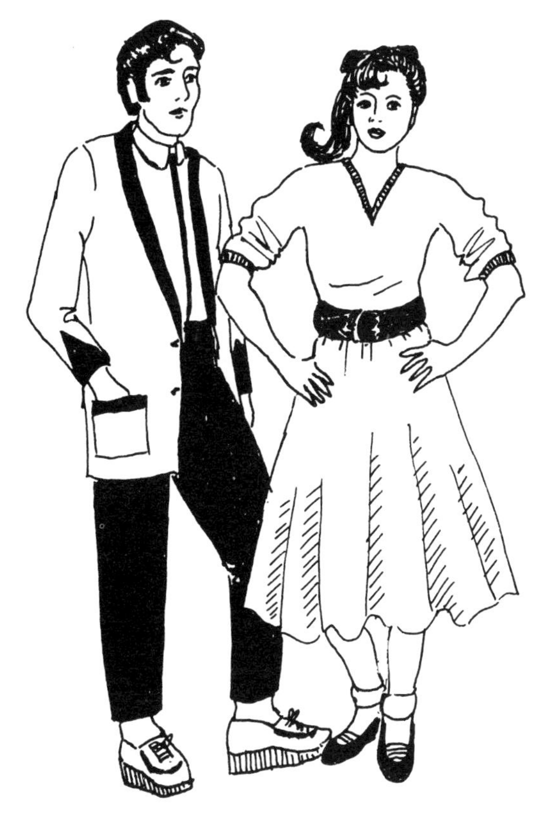

Fig. 4.69 'Teddy boy' and rock-'n'-roll image of the 1950s.

The Coronation of Queen Elizabeth II in 1953 sparked a 'look-a-like' phase.

A new focus in fashion highlighted the growing demand for youthful fashions. Young females as well as males had grown dissatisfied with wearing the same fashions as their parents. They suddenly demanded their own identity. This mood emerged in Paris, Britain and America in literature, fashions, music and films, which all expressed defiance, non-conformity and youthful optimism. In Paris this mood manifested itself as a new 'beat' generation. They held contemporary values in disregard and searched for a purpose in life. Their personal appearance was of little importance to them and the sloppy jumpers, tight trousers, unkempt long hair and jazz-crazy image reflected this. They were nicknamed the 'beatniks' (Fig. 4.68).

In Britain, although the beatnik image grew, it was also the teddy boy image that expressed youth culture, with carefully coiffured DA hair styles, three-quarter length jackets, drainpipe trousers and 'brothel-creeper' shoes (Fig. 4.69). In America it was James Dean and Marlon Brando who set the fashion with macho tee-shirts, leather jackets and denim jeans. The rock-n-roll upturned collar and swinging pelvis of Elvis Presley (Fig. 4.70) was an alternative.

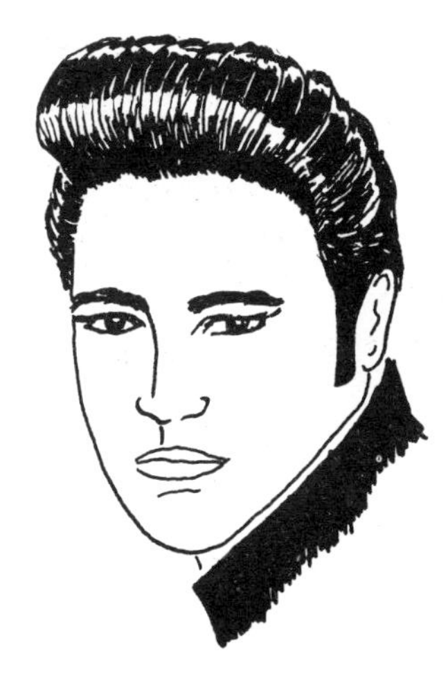

Fig. 4.70 The 'Elvis Presley' look.

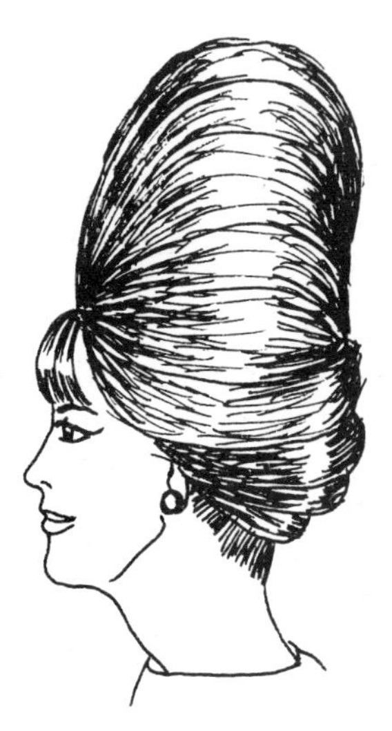

Fig. 4.71 'Bouffant' hair style.

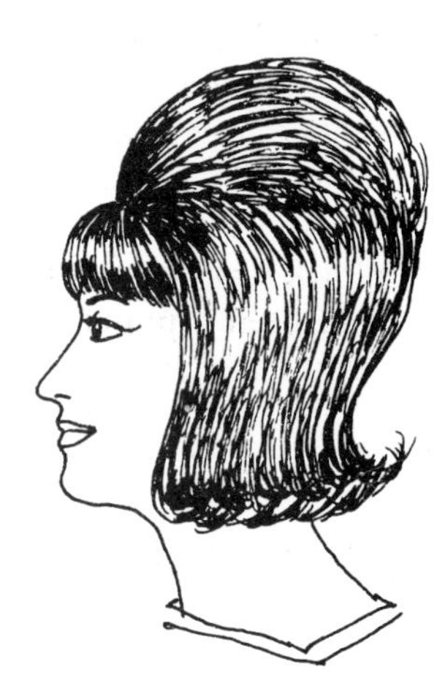

Fig. 4.72 'Bouffant' 'flick-up' style.

This new profitable market of the teenager switched the dominance of the fashion world from Paris and Italy to Britain. Art colleges started to produce new young British designers. One of them was Mary Quant, who opened up the first boutique selling only teenager fashions in 1955.

This search for youthful identity influenced hair fashions also. While mature women wore shorter, neater hair styles, the young experimented with back-combing. Although it was not a new technique and had been used discreetly along with false hair to gain enormous proportions of hair styles in the past, it was now being used blatantly on natural hair and being administered by the wearer's own hands. The styles started off on shorter

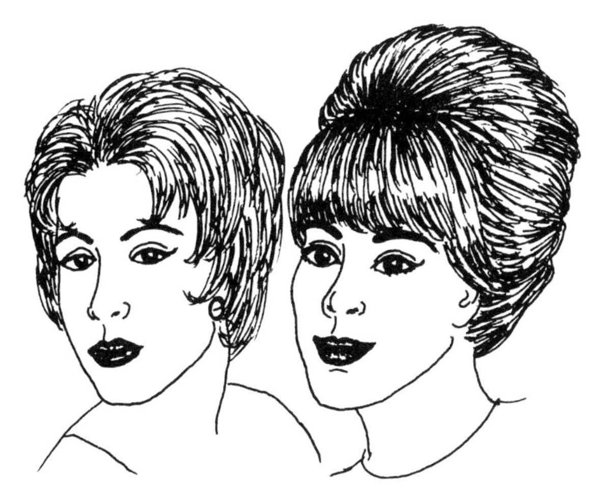

Fig. 4.73 The 1950s look.

hair with the back-combing used to gain volume, but towards the end of the decade the styles had grown to such heights that they resembled the unbalanced styles of the ancient Roman women, intended to be viewed only from the front (Fig. 4.71). Fringes were popular, and one of the most characteristic styles was a straight, long fringe with bouffant crown falling down into 'flick-ups' below the jaw line or lower (Fig. 4.72).

Rollers had been a popular invention and most women adopted them. It became a common sight to see roller-clad women in the streets, in shops and on public transport with their heads covered with a light scarf as a token of self-consciousness, but failing to conceal the mountainous landscape underneath. Use of cosmetics had been on the increase since the war. Max Factor and Rimmel were the most popular manufacturers of make-up at reasonable prices, so that most women could afford it. Lipstick in luscious, shiny reds was the most popular, and lips were the focus of the face, although an interest in the eyes emerged towards the end of the 1950s. Eyebrows were thick and well-shaped. Black eye-liner was worn discreetly, emphasising and shaping the eyes (Fig. 4.73).

1960–1970

In fashion the 1960s saw a breakdown in classic fashion rules. The swing from high couture Paris fashion to British boutique styles had started in the 1950s with Mary Quant. Now they took hold and there was an influx of small, dark, mysterious boutiques offering an alternative shopping experience to a select few. Canned music, strange boutique names and enthusiastic shop assistants suddenly made shopping a social event. The boutiques aimed towards the 15–25 age range and only offered limited sizes, basically because

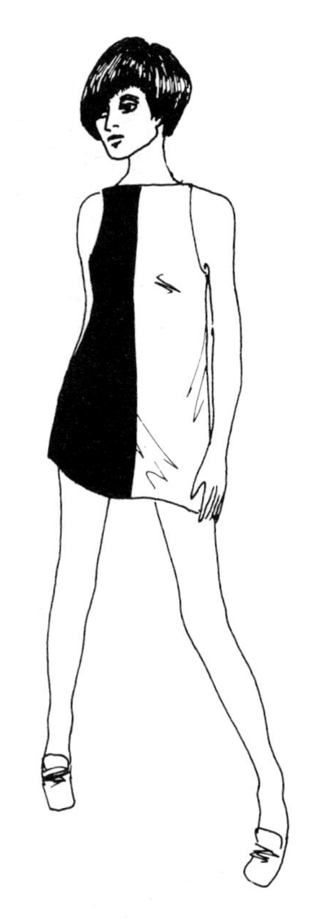

Fig. 4.74 The 'mini' dress by Mary Quant.

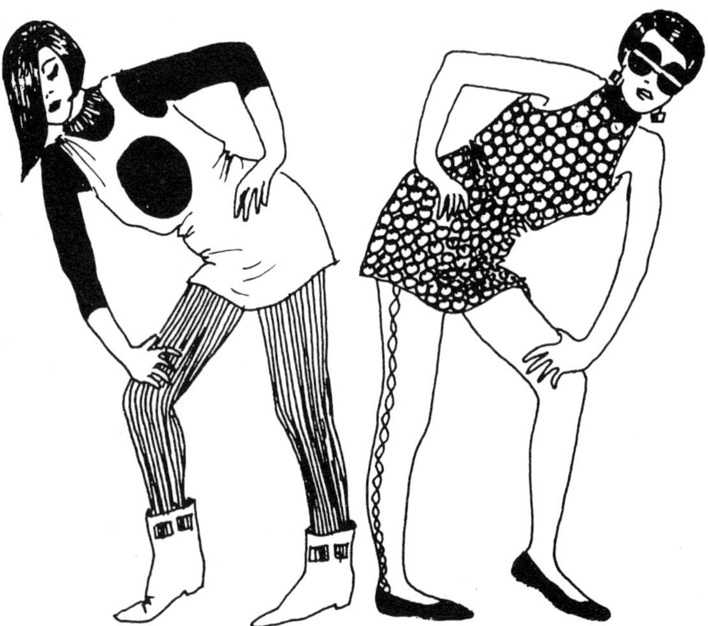

Fig. 4.75 1960s fashions inspired by current events – space travel, pop and op art.

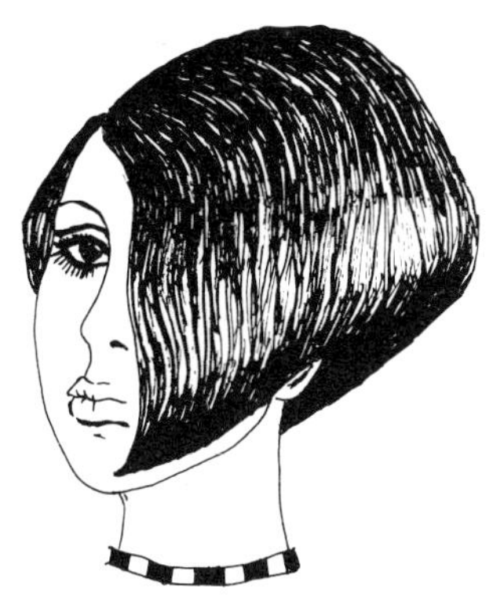

Fig. 4.76 Sassoon's variation on the classic bob.

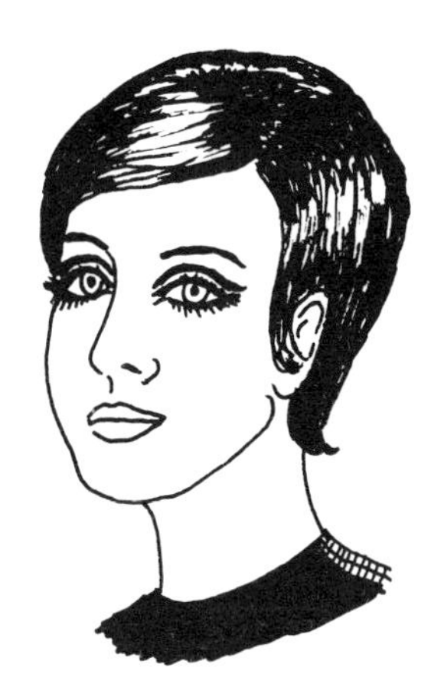

Fig. 4.77 Sassoon's 'garconne' style.

the new fashions desired a slim figure, not dissimilar to the look of the 1920s 'flapper' styles.

One of the most characteristic fashions of the 1960s was Mary Quant's mini (Fig. 4.74), which has been in the wings ever since, reappearing now and again in some revamped style. The hemlines of the 1920s had shocked; now these minis of the 1960s rose to astonishing heights, revealing as much thigh as possible without becoming indecent. Designers were also inventive with the use and combinations of new materials in their fashions: wool, paper, plastics, lurex and metals. They also dealt with current issues, such as space travel, pop and op art, and anti-war slogans (Fig. 4.75). This revolution in fashions reached through to the Paris fashion houses and some of their young, talented designers broke free. In particular, Yves St Laurent opened up his own Rive Gauche shops, and responded to the voice of youth.

Another revolution took place in the 1960s in hair styling. A young East End-trained hairdresser, Vidal Sassoon, popularised the trend of cutting and blow-drying the hair into style rather than laboriously setting, combing-out and lacquering. He created a range of styles that relied on precision cutting to create the shape and style. All that was needed afterwards was to wash the hair and blow-dry it (Fig. 4.76), which was also a unique method of hair styling. He revamped and popularised the old 1920s bob and was seen to work hand-in-hand with fashion designers to complement the fashions and help produce 'the look'. The prime example of this amalgamation was the creation of Twiggy, who became the face of the 1960s (Fig. 4.77). Twiggy's long, skinny, boyish figure became the desired shape as did her face. The pale, languid complexion enhanced by white lipstick was a stark contrast to the heavy black doe-like eyes. The look was then completed by Sassoon's short 'garçonne' or geometric hair style.

An alternative style of fashion to Quant emerged in the mid-60s. Barbara Hulanicki had started off with a successful mail-order business, and then later opened a shop in Kensington called Biba. The dominant fashion colours

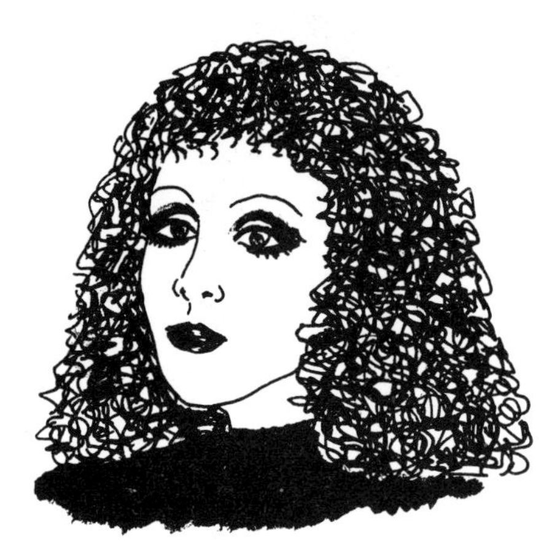

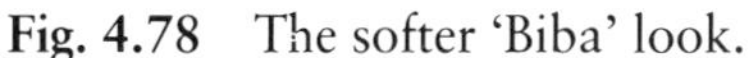

Fig. 4.78 The softer 'Biba' look.

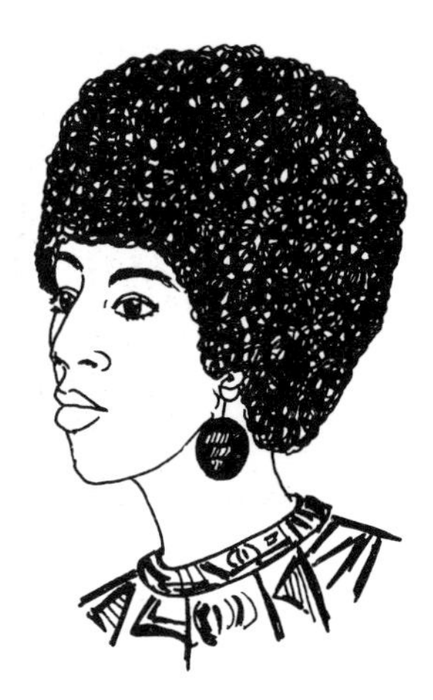

Fig. 4.79 Afro cut.

were black, plum and brown, and the style was vampish, glamorous and with a sense of mystery. Satin, silks and feather boas gave a hint of the Hollywood of the past (Fig. 4.78).

Another important advance was black fashion. Black models appeared for the first time in 1964. Up until this time black fashions had followed the trends of white ideals. A good example of this is the pop group, The Supremes, who wore straightened hair, wigs, make-up designed for white people and white fashions. In 1966 the Afro cut emerged (Fig. 4.79) and Black fashions became recognised in their own right, towards the end of the decade. 'Black is beautiful' was a well used phrase and black consciousness was slowly emerging. An interest in tribal hair styles produced an influx of fashionable black styles, in particular 'corn rowing' (Fig. 4.80) and Afro wigs, which were worn by both white and black males and females.

It was quite common for males and females to wear the same clothes, more often than not hipster bell-bottoms or 'loons' and 'grandad' vests, hence the name 'unisex' fashions.

1970–1980

After the intensity of the 1960s, the fashions and styles of the 1970s sought inspiration from nostalgia in an attempt to capture some kind of identity from the past. It seemed as though everybody was looking for a little niche that suited them, and consequently there was an assortment of different fashions all going on at the same time in a sort of chaotic fashion bonanza. From this mishmash developed an important progression in fashion styling, that of 'street fashion'. Ordinary people started to be the fashion innovators themselves, developing their own unique look rather than submitting to fashion designers.

The general mood, though, in the early 1970s was more romantic than

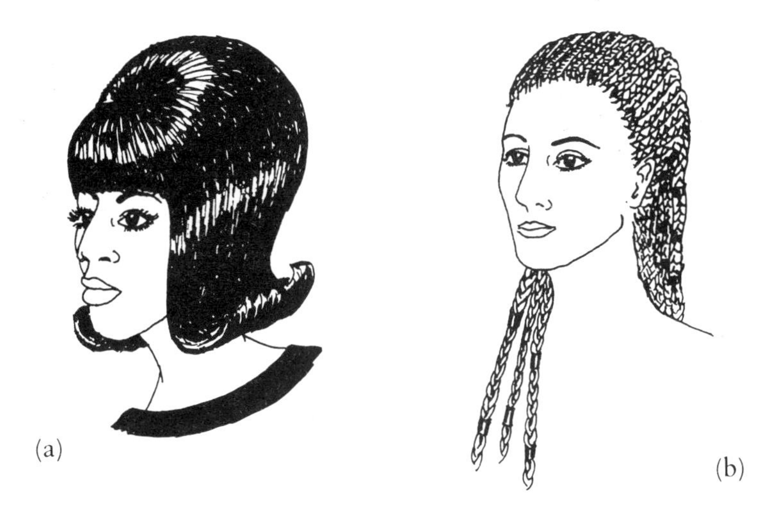

Fig. 4.80 (a) Black fashions imitated European styles in the 1960s; (b) then later a total reversal – European fashions imitated traditional black styles, e.g. the 'Bo Derek' look.

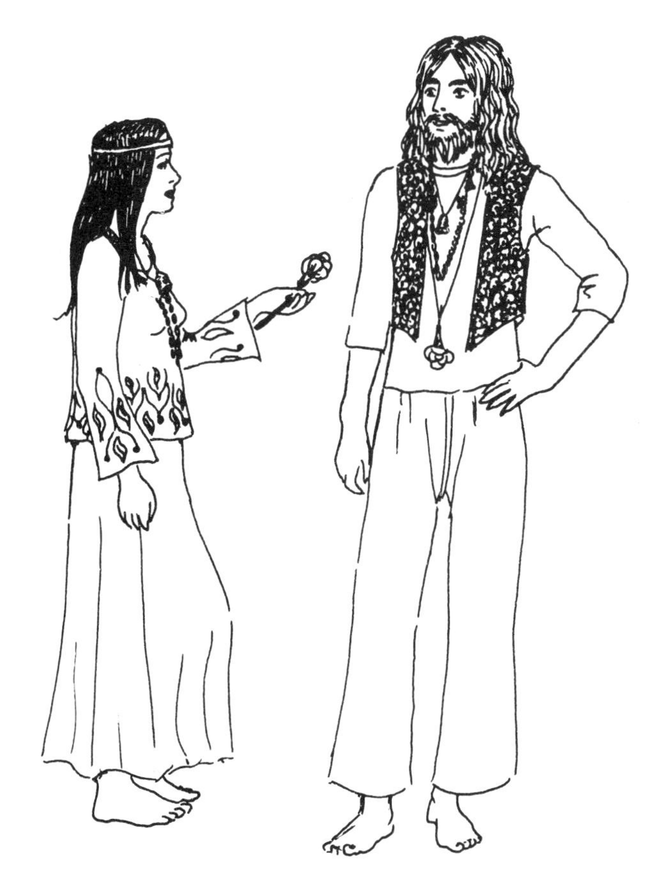

Fig. 4.81 Hippies.

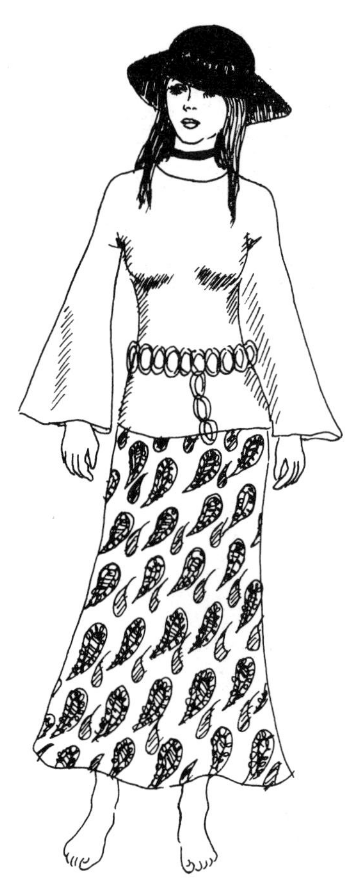

Fig. 4.82 The 'peasant' look.

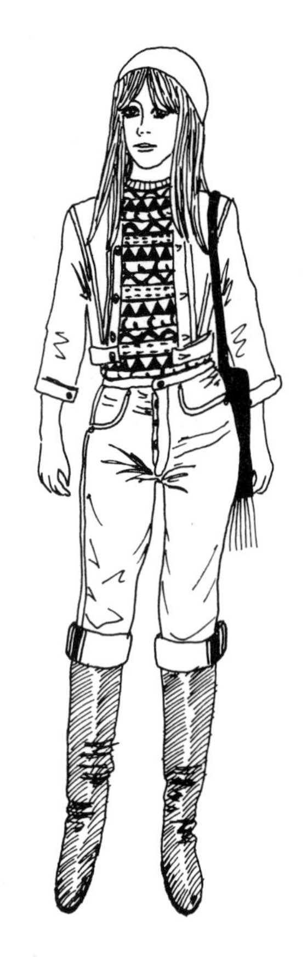

Fig. 4.83 The unisex 1970s look.

later, when it became more rebellious. The hippy cult hung on from the late 1960s. Their philosophy resembled that of the beatniks of the 1950s, and so did their appearance – plain, loose clothes, no shoes, long, unkept hair. They believed the spirit outshone material details, and their goal was world peace (Fig. 4.81). Other more romantic looks were: the peasant look promoted by Laura Ashley and Liberty prints (Fig. 4.82); the revival of 1930s clinging fashions along with platform shoes; the 1920s gangster moll Bonnie and Clyde look; hot pants; maxi clothes (which were inevitable as a reaction to the extreme '60s minis). The emancipated woman look returned with the popularity of trouser suits in bright colours, such as mauves, greens and mustards.

Black consciousness which had started in the 1960s now became a political force and was reflected in black fashions and hair styles. Ethnic fabrics and prints influenced white fashions. Tribal hair plaiting influenced the white hair styles and the 'Bo Derek' look emerged. Before, black fashions had always followed white fashions. Now the influence was reversed (Fig. 4.80).

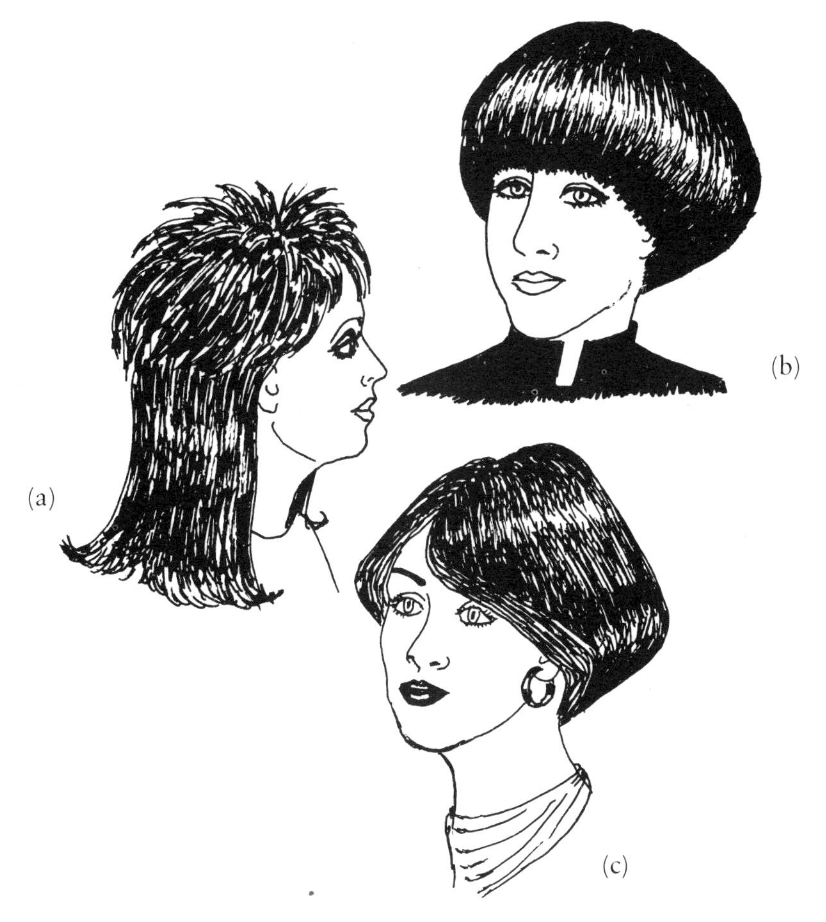

Fig. 4.84 1970s hair styles: (a) 'gypsy' cut; (b) 'Purdy' cut; (c) 'wedge'.

The punk movement was the most important fashion innovation of the late 1970s. The punk look was made popular by designer Vivienne Westwood and Malcolm McClaren. Punks aimed to shock and react against the social norm and establishment and they did this by wearing disturbing, threatening styles, materials and accessories – safety pins through their noses, chains, studs, bondage, plastic bags, straps, torn and shredded cloth (Fig. 4.85). The colours also reflected the mood: black and purple. The image was angry and vicious and was completed by severe heavy make-up and unconventional hair styles: bright green and pink mohicans, or short spiked hair that had been severely bleached and partially shaven. Punks boycotted hairdressers and instead created their outlandish styles by cutting and styling each other's hair or they did it themselves (see Fig. 4.86). From this rebellion, various hair salons sprang up such as Antenna, whose aim was solely to satisfy each individual client whether it was using conventional or unconventional methods. Colour was experimental, and the vivid shades were sometimes obtained by using carpet dyes or food colouring. The rigid texture of the

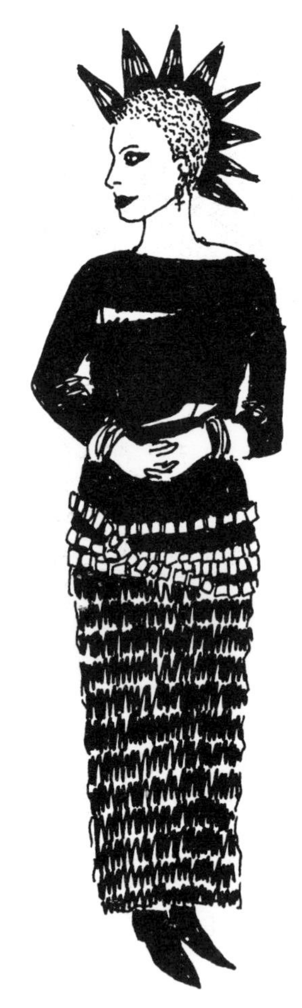

Fig. 4.85 Punk look.

outrageous styles was achieved by rubbing sugar or soap into the hair to begin with, but later hair manufacturers were quick to catch on and hair gel became widely used.

This movement was interesting because it was the first time that ordinary people actually had control over their own image instead of the fashion designer or stylist dictating it, and that street fashion actually influenced high fashion. Designers such as Zandra Rhodes and Jeff Banks took their inspiration from it and designed collections incorporating safety pins, bondage straps and deliberate rips and tears.

1980–1990

Gothic punk emerged as the older punk styles faded. The image was less severe but still shocked. Gothic punk still favoured black. Styles were longer

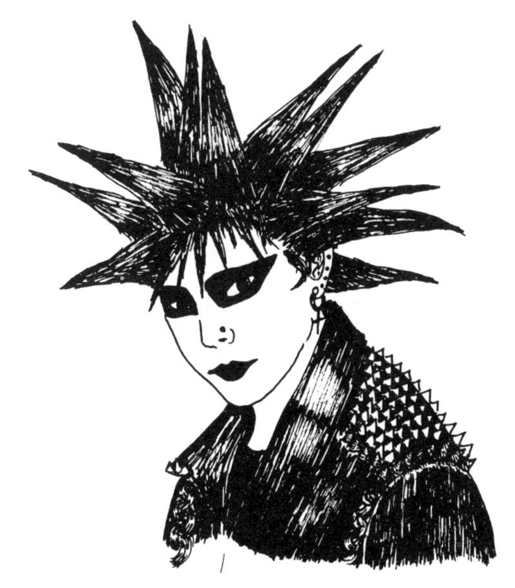

Fig. 4.86 Rebellious punk image.

with chains. Studded belts and crucifixes were worn as accessories. The hair styles incorporated very short sides with long layers over the rest of the head, back-combed and spiked out, and the make-up was still in heavy black and mauves but drawn more artistically (Fig. 4.87).

The punk movement had influenced fashion as a whole and the early 1980s saw punk become respectable. Fashions for all ages reflected some influence of punk, and in hair styles too, the prevalent use of gels, sprays and foams enabled all age groups to achieve the unkempt, windswept look. The vivid colouring also affected hair designs. Manufacturers produced a range of bright semi–permanent colours in pink, green and blue which might be put onto bleached hair; sometimes on the tips of the hair; or in a small area in the front or at the back or sides. Certain aspects of the punk fashions were accepted and interpreted into the current fashion trends. Trousers and jeans echoed the bondage image. Tee-shirts were sold supporting tears and holes. Accessories included pins, chains and straps.

In the early 1980s designers soon realised the influence of current pop groups on fashion trends. Along with the powerful vehicle of television, the groups became performing mannequins, selling new ideas and images to an extremely wide audience. Music and fashion became a strong weapon in the creation of new images. One of the designers to utilise this capacity was Vivienne Westwood. She created the new 'romantic look' which was best illustrated by groups such as Spandau Ballet, and the 'pirate' look pioneered and modelled by Adam Ant.

Another strong influence on the fashion scene in the late 1970s and early 1980s came from America. The increasing popularity of jogging, keep-fit and sports brought the trend for jogging suits, sweatshirts, work-out kits,

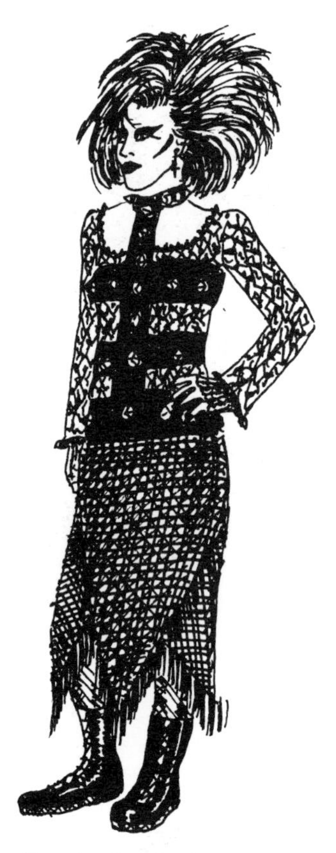

Fig. 4.87 Gothic punk.

leotards, footless tights, and trainers (Fig. 4.88). Sporting clothes also influenced street fashion. Ski pants became popular worn with high-heels in such colours as bright orange, yellows and lime green.

Over the last three or four years fashions have still been dominated by street fashions, although they have tended to be gimmicky – fluorescent colours, hip-hop and acid house crazes appealed to the young while the popularity of wearing black was favoured by the more mature age group and took quite a while to die out. There has also been a strong influence of African prints interpreted into Western fashions (Fig. 4.89).

4.12 FASHION TRENDS IN THE EARLY 1990s

Fashions in the 1990s, it seems, have sought for an identity. Some have reflected back in time for inspiration, such as the revival of the 1960s space-age look and also an attempt to revive the 1970s hippy fashions. Others have focused on the future and concocted fashions as individual as they can be, such as surreal or futuristic looking brassieres worn as tops. It

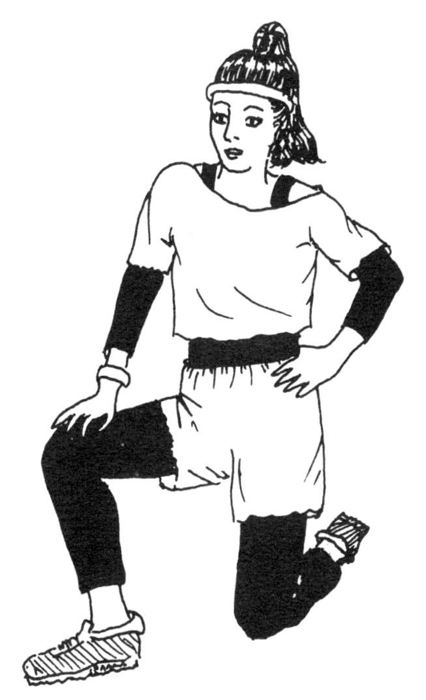

Fig. 4.88 American 'jogging' influence on fashion.

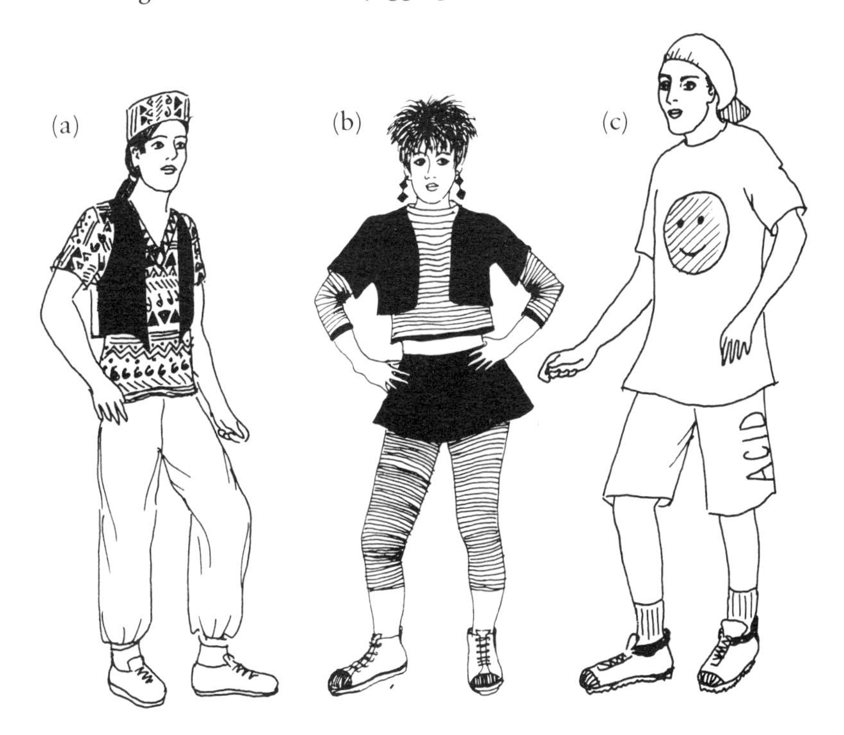

Fig. 4.89 Late 1980s street fashions: (a) African influence; (b) sporty 'mini' look; (c) 'acid house' fashions.

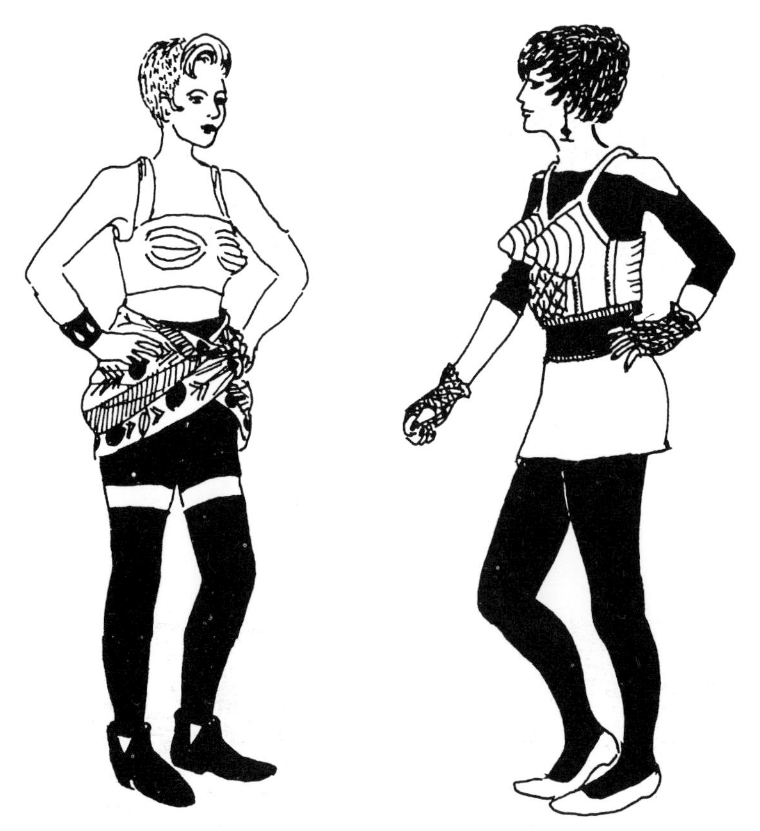

Fig. 4.90 Surreal and futuristic influence on fashion.

still seems that the fashion-conscious youth have not yet got over the thrill of shocking (Fig. 4.90).

One of the more important campaigns of the 1990s that has affected fashion is the Green issue. Concern for the environment and the constant depleting of resources has resulted in fabrics being made 'environmentally friendly'. Also, cosmetics and hair products have been affected by this issue. Substances harmful to the environment have been removed and replaced by more natural ingredients, and indeed the testing of these products on animals has also been seen, quite rightly, as unnecessary and cruel.

Hair styling in the 1990s

Hair styles around today reflect the variations of different lifestyles and images. Although modifications of the bob have been a predominant feature in fashionable styles (Fig. 4.91), so too has the punky approach to adding body and volume to the hair (Fig. 4.92) although these styles are much more tame than those of the 1970s. Short, cropped hair styles have become popular

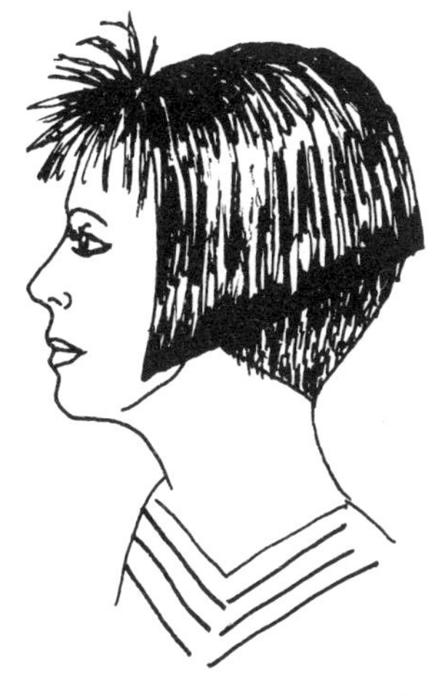

Fig. 4.91 Modified 1960s bob cut.

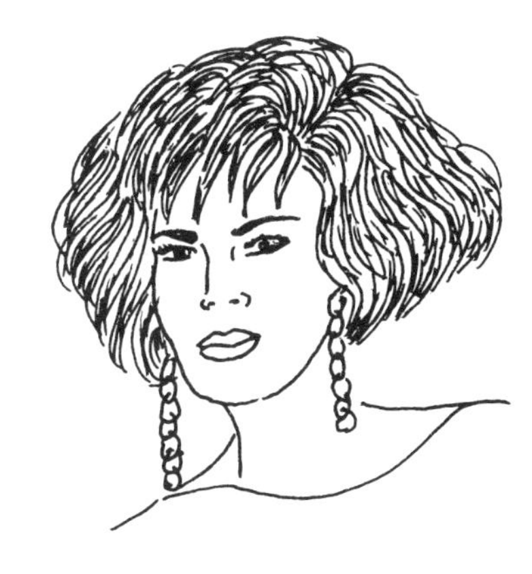

Fig. 4.92 Style influenced by punk.

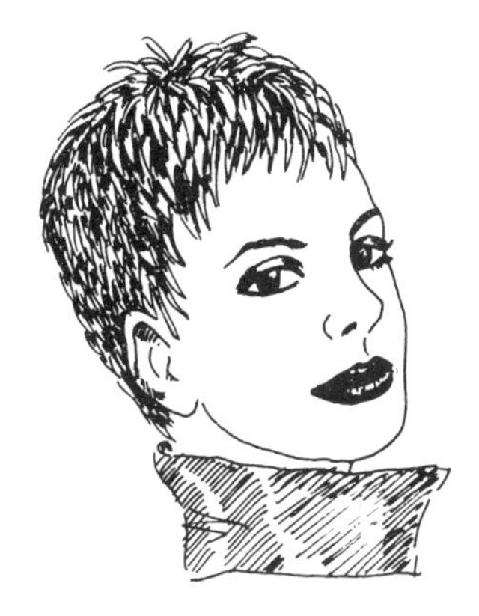

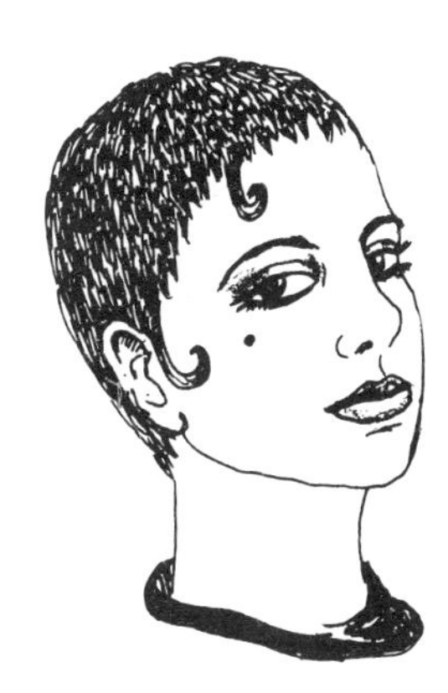

Fig. 4.93 Short textured hair styles of the early 1990s.

too, either with a windswept appearance or sleek, smooth and wet looking. Both styles are attained with the aid of gels or sprays. Sometimes the cropped hair is severely bleached, and then gel applied, resulting in a very textural effect (Fig. 4.93).

Extensions on both black and white hair have also become a common sight. False hair is woven into the natural hair resulting in an abundance of tight plaits (Fig. 4.94). Men's hair styles also vary. The popularity for a small pigtail at the nape of the neck that was a favourite in the late 1970s and early 1980s has made a modified come-back (see Fig. 4.95). A preference for longer hair, tied back into a pony-tail, has also become popular in certain sections of the male population. These are not necessarily old hippies; it is a common sight to see smart businessmen with their hair carefully coiffured into a neat pony-tail too.

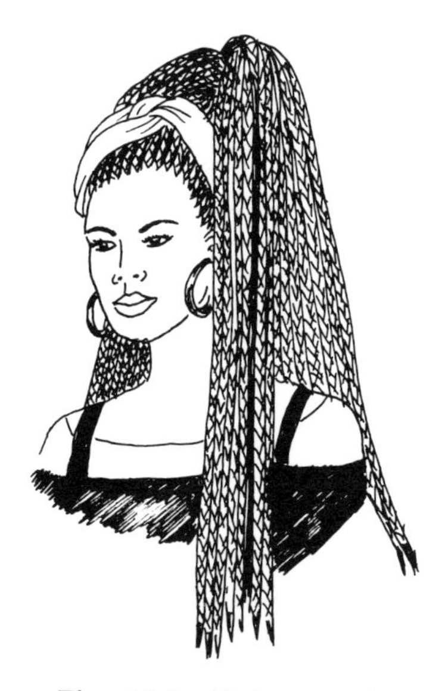

Fig. 4.94 Hair extensions.

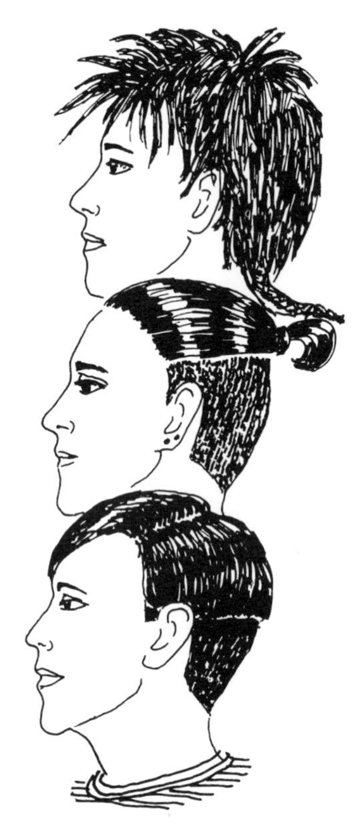

Fig. 4.95 Men's hair styles of the early 1990s.

Another trend in men's hair styling is a variation on the short back and sides, with a blatant line cut around the back of the head. This style is a favourite with children as well.

The aftermath of punk is still felt in some of the men's styles which give a disarrayed appearance.

5

Salon Design

Most hair stylists would like to run their own businesses eventually. This would give them the opportunity to combine their creative ideas, talent, business skills and ambition, so that their new salon becomes stamped with their individual mark. In order to achieve this ambition it is important to observe a few basic design points:

(1) Create a clear image which is targeted at the right section of the public.
(2) Ensure that this image is right for the particular location.
(3) Give the premises a professional 'look'.
(4) Make sure you deliver the same quality of service that you advertise.

For our purpose we will deal with the two areas of salon design separately, i.e. exteriors and interiors.

5.1 EXTERIORS

The first impression a prospective client has of the salon is its facade or front. This is the salon's first important selling point because it can either entice clients inside or deter them.

Here are a few fundamental questions that need to be considered:

Who do you want to appeal to? Is it a cross-section of the public, young and old? Or just a certain section such as the young or fashionable?

Is the image that you are aiming for clear, firstly to you and then the public?

Is the image you are considering suitable for the area? For instance, it might not be financially viable to go for a fashionable, trendy image in an area that is populated predominantly by the elderly.

Does the structure and layout of the front of the salon suit the image? For instance, if the salon is above a butcher's shop it could be difficult to appear flamboyant or exclusive.

Does the name of the salon suit the image you are aiming at? For instance, a salon aiming at the young and fashionable might not be best presented by a name such as 'Doreen's'.

Does the style of lettering or graphics used suit the name? Consider the shape and size of the letters, whether they are bold capitals or fine handwriting, or if they are to be set horizontally across the front of the window or diagonally to one side, and also consider the use of other media, such as neon.

What colour scheme would best present the right image? Black and white gives a clean contrast, whereas the use of gold or silver might suggest a touch of glamour.

Is the image accessible? To strike the right balance of creating an image that gives a sense of exclusiveness but still appears approachable can be a challenge.

Does the image of the salon suit the rest of the architecture surrounding it? Too often salons totally ignore the possible design features of the building that could be enhanced and extended into the design of the shop.

All these questions and options should be considered before the right image can be clearly defined. The question about appealing to the public or certain sections of the public can be a tricky one. At the end of the day whatever your ideals are you have to make money to survive and limiting your clientele can mean taking a chance. Some salons strike a good balance by offering perms and sets only on certain days to entice older clients.

Window displays

The next step to consider is the window display, and this should be well thought out.

It is important to consider what you intend to do with the window. If your intentions are to put in a display (hair products, photographs, etc.) then think of the best way to arrange it considering the window space. If you intend the window to be a part of the whole exterior design, then it should blend in well with the surroundings. But beware, some salons that have chosen this feature have actually gone over-the-top and become *too* exclusive, so that the public are unaware that they are hairdressing salons. This might be because there was no evidence in the window, especially if the window had tinted glass, or in some cases it might be that the salon name (which is usually the giveaway) was too exclusive so there was no indication that the shop's ware was hair! Instead it could easily have been an insurance broker or such like.

Generally speaking, though, people are more interested in an unusual or attractive window presentation, which also suggests an individual approach

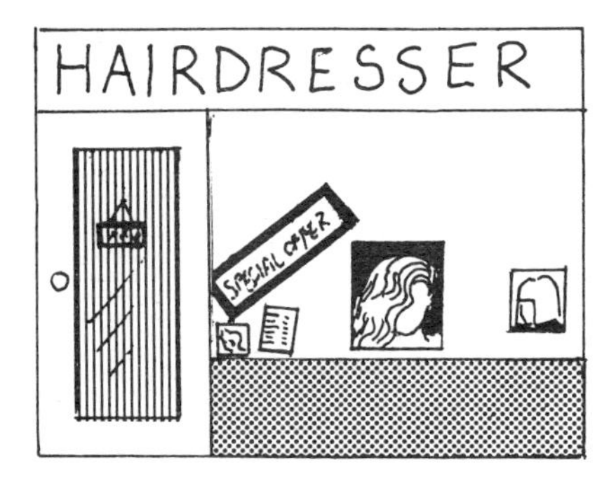

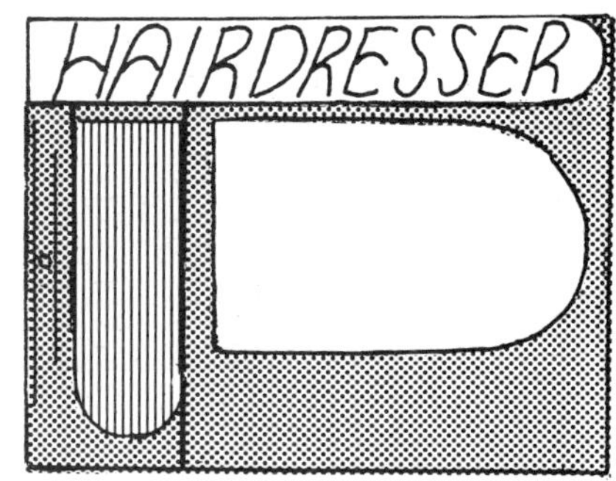

Fig. 5.1 Window presentations. The shop on the left suggests confusion, whereas the shop on the right incorporates the whole front as part of the design, suggesting an individual and interesting approach.

by the stylists inside. A disorganised or tatty window display, on the other hand, suggests that a similar attitude or treatment prevails inside (see Fig. 5.1) and acts as an effective deterrent for any prospective clients.

If you are considering using a window display there are some important points to consider first. The most important is that whatever display you decide on should incorporate the whole window area, and be a total design. The theme of the window should flow, whether it is a display of photographs, a colour theme or a more atmospheric creation. The line and balance of the design will determine the fluency of the display, whether the display is arranged to a horizontal, vertical or diagonal format, or whether it is simulating a square, circle or triangle. Whatever the design, it should be clear and consistent (see Figs 5.2–5.4).

If photographs are used then they should all be of a similar quality and radiate a degree of professionalism. Photographs of styles actually created in the salon will enhance the salon's credibility. If commercial photographs of hair styles are used then make sure that the stylists' skills match those that are being displayed. Also make the gesture of updating the styles that are on display occasionally – it deadens any incentive to see a row of faded old photographs.

The more interesting salon fronts are those that tend to be a bit more imaginative and follow some type of theme (Fig. 5.5). For instance, some salons are able to change their display according to the seasons or indeed to illustrate current trends such as the Green issue or nostalgia. It need not be costly and shows a willingness to change and a desire to be different.

Be aware of the potential of the salon front and fully utilise it as it will blatantly reflect the attitude to the work that goes on inside. If the shop window looks tatty and has not been changed for years then it strongly suggests that the same has happened to the stylists inside – that they are locked away in some time-warp, totally ignorant of the changing world around them.

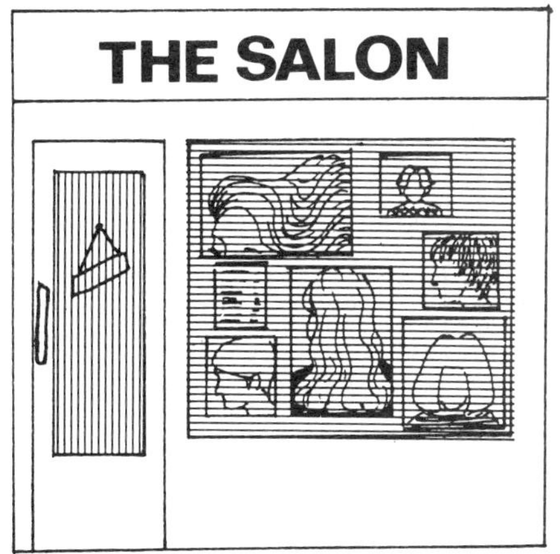

Fig. 5.2 Too much information and too many images in the window result in confusion and look messy.

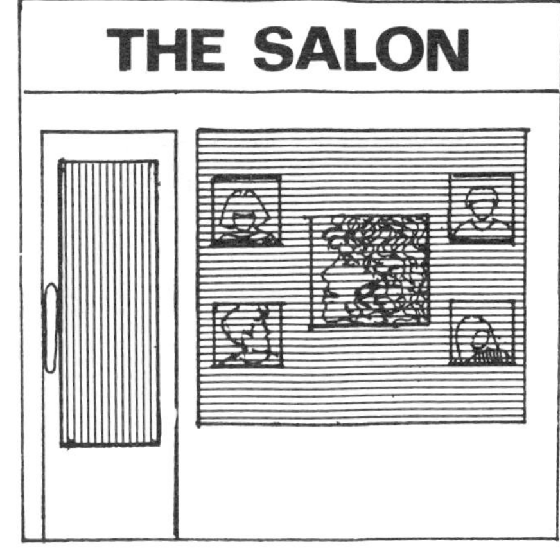

Fig. 5.3 A symmetrical use of photographs in the window suggests an organised salon and adds a touch of professionalism.

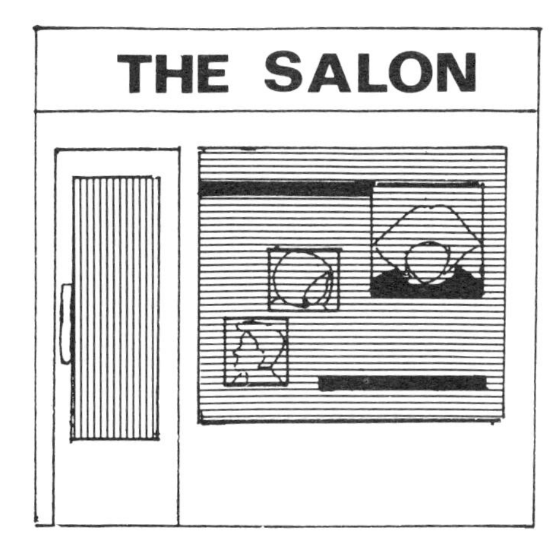

Fig. 5.4 An asymmetrical use of the window suggests individuality and can appear interesting.

Another point that should be considered is the use of notices in the window. All too often a good salon display has been disfigured by a makeshift notice advertising special offers, or requesting models, juniors or stylists. We will cover the use of lettering in more depth in Chapter 6 on Advertising. It is possible, if you have the aptitude, to make your own notices adequately, but as an alternative commercially printed notices are available from wholesale hairdressing suppliers.

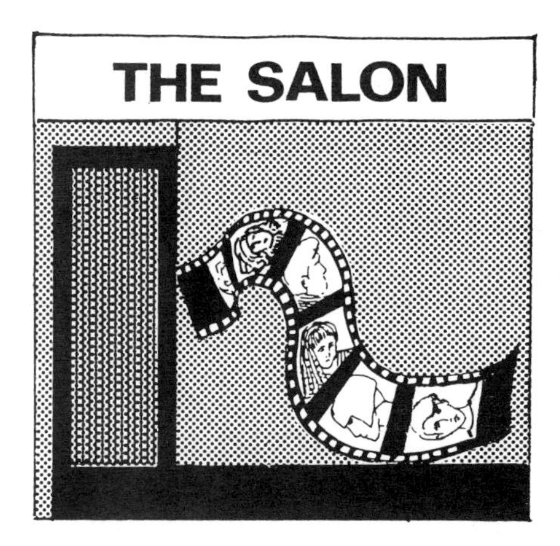

Fig. 5.5 The most interesting salon fronts tend to be unusual and imaginative.

5.2 INTERIORS

Once you have enticed the client into the salon, she should find that the interior lives up to the image you have projected from the outside. The design of the salon interior should consider the clients' needs primarily, and aim to create a comfortable and secure environment. At the same time you must recognise the importance of the creative and spontaneous elements that make the hairdressing salon such an interesting and lively place.

It was all the rage in the 1960s and 70s to offer unisex hairdressing salons where both sexes sat side by side while their hair was being shampooed, permed or styled. During the 1980s and since there has been more of a move towards accommodating the different sexes in separate areas, although they might still be under the same roof. The general mood is that men and women while having hairdressing treatments feel more comfortable with their own kind, so many salons are wisely acknowledging this current move and offering separate services in the same salon, for example, with women upstairs and men downstairs or splitting the salon into two areas on the same level. The important feature to recognise here is that most women will have different preferences to most men about the design of the interiors. I think it would be true to say that men would feel more comfortable in an interior that was designed for them rather than having to share a predominantly feminine environment.

One of the most important points to observe when designing the interior of any salon is that the inside needs to be considered as a whole. The design that is finally agreed upon must flow throughout. All too often salon interiors suffer a style confusion, mixing different styles of furniture, fittings and decor, so that the overall result is a mishmash, appears messy and is not very professional-looking. The rule is to keep it simple and consistent to look most effective and professional. Here are some different ways of achieving a simple co-ordinated look effectively without any confusion:

(1) Use a repeated motif or pattern.
(2) Use the same shape for chairs, mirrors, units and so on, maybe an angular shape or a rounded shape (see Figs 5.6 and 5.7).
(3) If you are going to use different styles of furniture make sure there are no more than two and that they do complement one another. If needs be get expert advice first.
(4) Use colour co-ordination, choosing perhaps two or three colours that run throughout the whole salon interior on the walls, floor, ceiling, furniture, equipment, etc.

Many professional salon design companies are available, so use them. Some have showrooms where you can go and see examples of interior ideas, many have free catalogues which will offer different themes and illustrate the different materials available, and most will offer expert consultations without any obligation. Use them all to get a good range of ideas and examples of the possibilities available for your salon interior. If you decide to put the interior of your salon into the hands of one of these companies, make sure your ideas, if you have any, are heard and certainly incorporated into the final overall plans. All too often the designer seems to take over, so remember, *you* are the expert, *you* have to work there. Last but not least, remember *you* have to pay for the work so make sure you know precisely how much it is going to cost *before* any work begins.

If you wish to design the interior yourself, make sure that you have a clear idea of the image you want beforehand. Make detailed plans, depicting the colour scheme, the choice of materials, e.g. wood, steel etc., the shape and design of the furnishings and fittings, and all other details, such as flooring, shelving, reception area. When you have an overall impression, get advice as to whether it works as a design or not.

Before you finally decide on any of the designs for a new interior it would be wise to observe a few practical suggestions:

(1) When choosing furnishings, etc., always go for quality rather than cheaper alternatives, as the quality products will be more durable and maintain a good appearance as they age. The cheaper furnishings might look great for a short while but they will soon look scruffy, and will need replacing far sooner.
(2) Make sure you choose all the major expensive equipment, such as styling units, chairs, dryers, wash basins, reception desk, etc., in neutral colours. Then you can afford to choose, perhaps, the less expensive items such as towels, gowns, wall and ceiling decoration, in more definite colours or designs. This will allow you to change the overall look of the salon interior from time to time by changing the colour scheme of these items without any major expense.
(3) Practicality is a key point to consider. The design of the salon interior

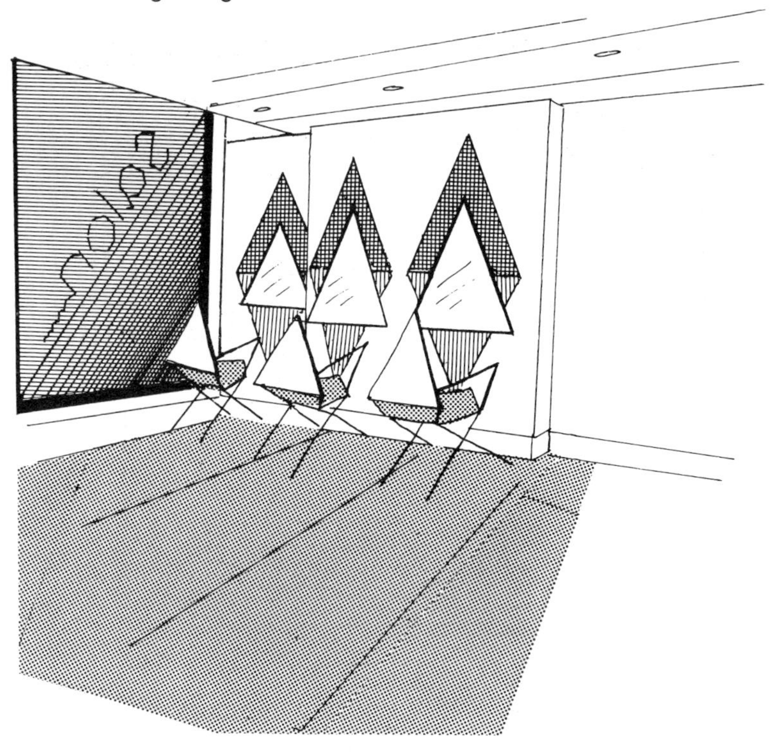

Fig. 5.6 Achieving a co-ordinated look by using a consistent shape throughout – geometric shapes.

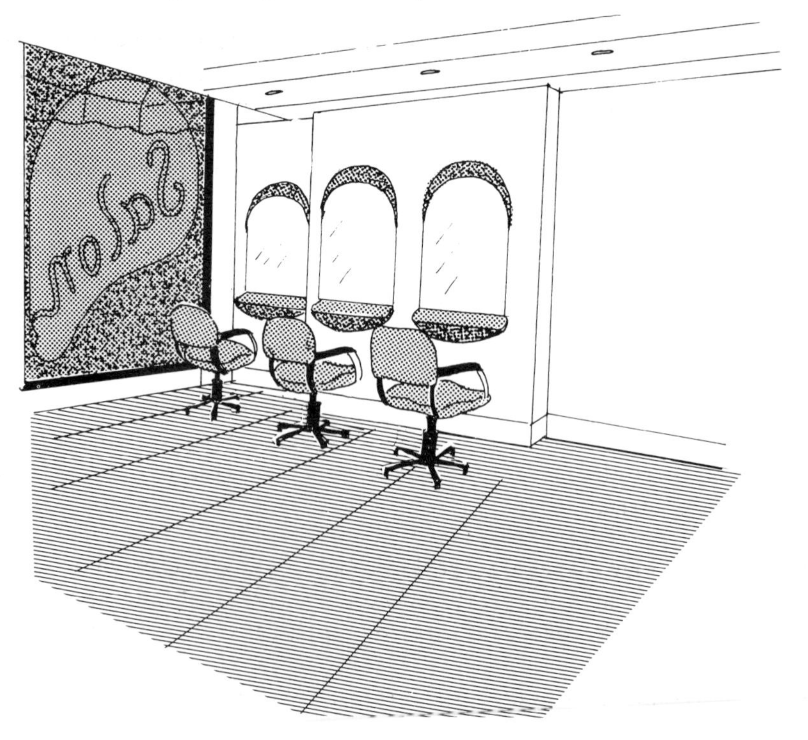

Fig. 5.7 Contrast of same interior using rounded shapes.

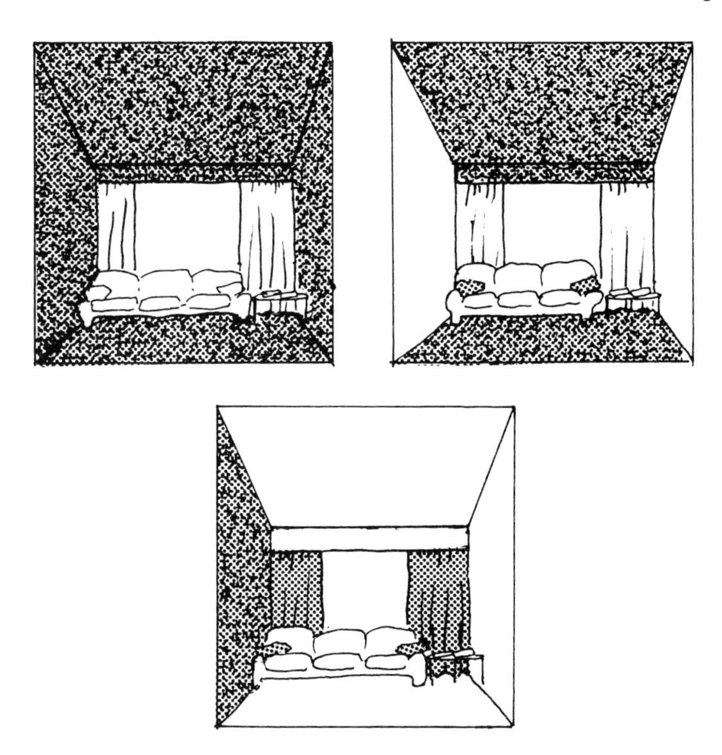

Fig. 5.8 Use of colour affecting the apparent size of the room.

has to be dealt with realistically. For instance, carpet throughout might just be the right ingredient to finish the decor off so it looks splendid, but the chemical processes, and the amount of cut hair involved in hairdressing would ruin the effect quickly, so it would be more appropriate to choose a floor surface that would cope, such as linoleum tiles.

Points to consider when designing salon interiors

(1) Creating space

This must be the most important point to consider – the necessity to create space within the interior, unless you are fortunate enough to have acquired premises that match thc Albert Hall! There are a number of different ways to create a sense of space:

- Choice of colour. Generally speaking, bold strong intense colours will make the room appear smaller, while paler tones will add space. The combination of the two can affect the apparent size of the room (see Fig. 5.8).
- Careful lay-out of furniture. Make sure all the corners and alcoves are

not wasted and are utilised to the full. The wall space of the salon probably far exceeds the floor space, so use it as much as you can. Mounted shelving, cupboards or units can be stacked on top of each other instead of sitting side by side.

- Use of mirrors. It can also become quite a feature if they are strategically placed so an image seems to go on infinitely.

(2) The use of colour

Colour can be used to create a suitable atmosphere, as we have mentioned in Chapter 2. Our emotional responses to different colours vary, so it would be wise to check the atmosphere you want before deciding on a colour scheme. For instance, a salon painted a bold colour such as a red or mauve might overpower the client and make her feel extremely uncomfortable, whereas a salon painted predominantly black or brown might make the client feel dowdy and dismal.

The temperature evoked by the colour is also important to consider. A salon painted in a cool blue might be heaven in the heat of the summer, but first thing in the morning, or in the middle of winter it will feel extremely cold.

Colours, like fashion trends, tend to change in popularity, so while it might be tempting to have the salon painted in the current fashionable colour, unless you intend to have it redecorated every six months, it will soon look dated. Generally speaking, it would be wise to choose more of a neutral colour or just a hint of colour and then create more of a colourful atmosphere by adding photographs, plants and other wall decorations.

(3) The use of pattern and texture

The use of pattern can be an effective way of creating an atmosphere and making the salon visually interesting. Repetitive wall patterns, positive and negative shapes, or even a wall mural or graffiti wall can add an interesting feature to the decoration. Textural effects on the walls, ceiling or floor can also enhance an interior and give it unusual qualities. Texture can be used along with colour or lighting to create an interesting environment.

(4) The use of lighting

The choice of lighting is important in the salon and there are many varieties available, depending on the effect or atmosphere you want to create in your interior. Some salons have adopted the combination of low voltage lighting running throughout, with spotlights in appropriate places, such as styling, cutting and colouring areas, to give maximum visibility. Other salons have opted to use halogen lights throughout. These give a natural daylight effect, which is excellent for colouring work.

The use of coloured lights in the interior, which was mentioned to some extent in Chapter 2, should be approached with caution. A coloured light will affect the colour of everything it falls upon (including hair and skin!), so a *green* chair in your salon interior under a *red* light will appear *black*. Beware, not only will it change your colour scheme, it will also affect the colour of your clients' hair, making colour treatments difficult. Who knows what colour combinations could be walking out of the salon door!

(5) Other effective features to consider

There are different features that salons can offer to increase their individuality, which can be a good selling point. For instance, some salons have come to an arrangement with the local art gallery to exhibit local artists' paintings and sculptures, which are also for sale. The clever thing about this is that they can be changed quite frequently. Other salons have video monitors which have a double purpose. They can be used for staff-training purposes and they can offer clients pop videos, fashion shows etc.

Plants are another important feature worth mentioning for salon interiors as they are extremely versatile. They create a wonderful healthy atmosphere; they are very decorative; they can be used to echo the predominant shapes in the salon, sharp and angular, or soft and rounded; and they can be used to screen off an area.

Remember, preferences for interior decoration are as varied as people themselves, so if the opportunity arises for you to design a salon, then as long as you have a clear idea of the image you desire and you feel confident it is right, go for it.

6

Advertising

Advertising and promotion are powerful media, and good or bad advertising can determine the success of a product regardless of its quality. Certain advertising techniques are more effective than others, and it tends to be the novel and unusual methods that are eye-catching and get results.

In the salon, advertising skills need to be employed in promoting products, services and skills. Attractive displays, eye-catching visual advertisements, such as photographs, as well as neat notices are all methods available, but the most effective method of selling a service or product is through the stylists themselves. Hairdressers should, because of the nature of their work, possess some salesmanship skills. They are the experts in their field and should be able to sell a product if they believe it is good. Clarity and honesty are the best attributes that should be employed when promoting, as they will instil respect and confidence in the prospective client.

Displays in the salon should observe the rules of successful advertising as well as retaining a level of balance and proportion. If, for instance, a new perm is being promoted in the salon, a stacked pyramid of the product in a corner might look good against the decor, but it will give no information about the product and will give the salon the appearance of a supermarket. A combination of visual and written information concerning the product, along with an arrangement that is attractive to the eye would be more successful. In advertising the written information acts as the core, transmitting all the relevant points of sale, whilst the visual picture explains, simplifies and creates an image around the product. This combination is a forceful mix and consequently affects us all, one way or the other.

An advertisement must be complete and consistent. If a theme is used it must flow throughout. If wording is used it must be clear. Whichever theme is employed, one thing is sure: *it must relate to the product or service being advertised* if it is to be effective.

Large visual advertisements, particularly for products, are usually supplied by the manufacturers themselves, but how and where they are displayed is

(a) 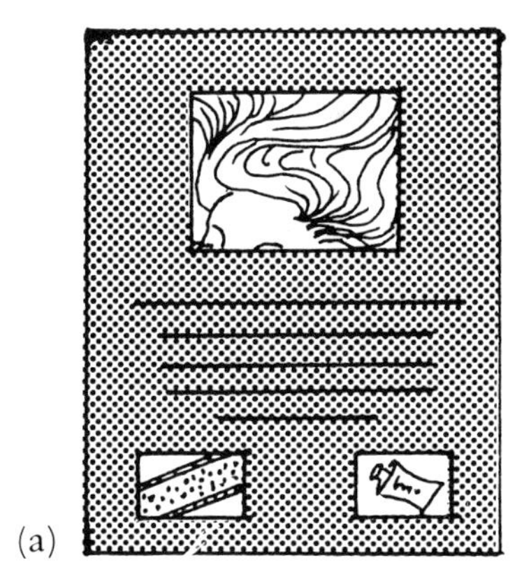 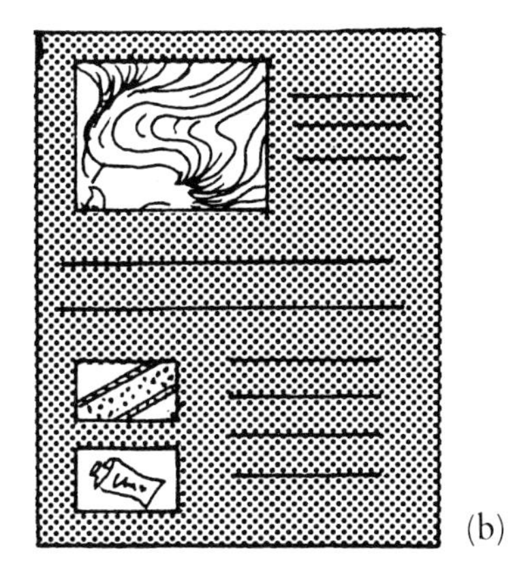 (b)

Fig. 6.1 Contrast of lay-outs: (a) symmetrical; (b) asymmetrical.

usually left up to the salon. This material can be presented in an exciting or imaginative way, or can be made to look very dull, and it does not need much imagination to work out which would be the most successful.

Special offers are among the most common notices displayed on salon windows, alongside models required notices. Although these are available commercially, a basic understanding of lay-out and lettering will enable salons to produce good results themselves.

6.1 LAY-OUT

The basic rules to remember for lay-out are:

(1) The purpose of the design should be well defined.
(2) The lay-out should be kept as simple as possible.
(3) Whatever technique is used, a harmonious theme or a contrast of images, the result should work as a whole concept.

The lay-out must adhere to the principles of basic design (see Chapter 1) as the harmony between the written material and visual representation, if used, is an important issue. There are many rules and regulations concerning the dos and don'ts of professional lay-out and advertising, but for our purpose we only need to concern ourselves with a few:

(1) Symmetrical and asymmetrical compositions can be used to gain different results (See Fig. 6.1).
(2) Choose appropriate colours to represent the right mood. If you want an element of sophistication then opt for black and gold. For a fun-loving fashionable look opt for a selection of brighter colours, e.g. pinks, greens, or yellows. For a feeling of mystery choose mauves, blacks or purples.

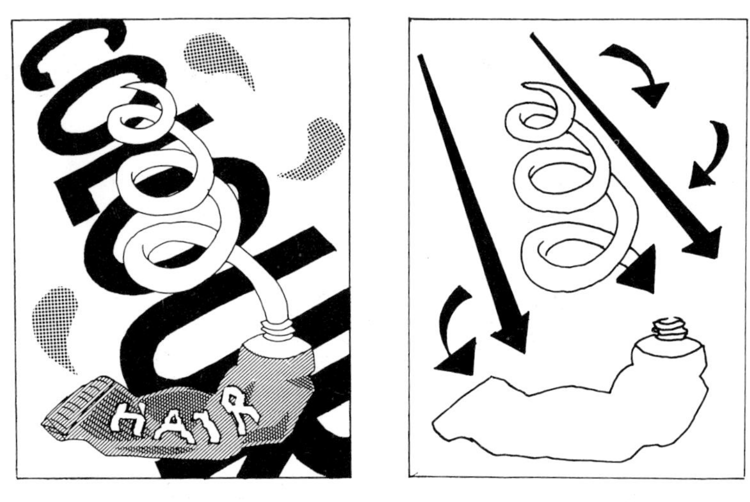

Fig. 6.2 Leads into the picture help to focus on the product.

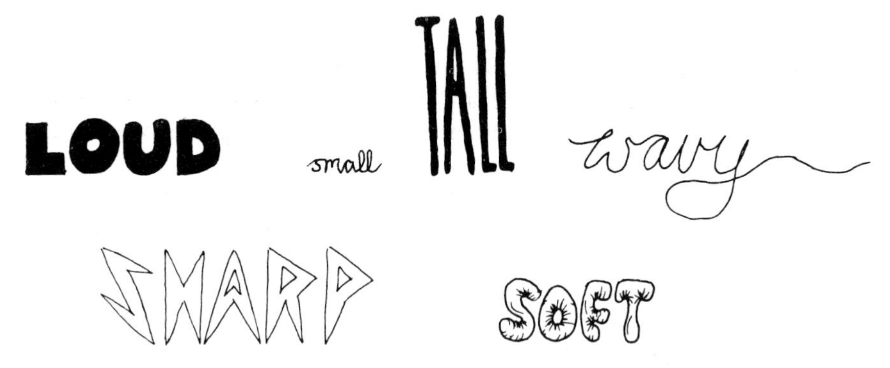

Fig. 6.3 Examples of expressive lettering.

(3) Remember that the eye will generally read a picture as it does a book, starting from the top, left hand corner. You may need to place obvious leads into the picture, such as arrows or lines, so that your main image or message dominates (See Fig. 6.2).

6.2 LETTERING

The use of lettering is as important as the lay-out. The size, shape and character of the letters will evoke a certain feeling, much the same as different lines can evoke different ideas (See Fig. 6.3). It is important to be aware of the possibilities of different letterings and the 'feelings' they convey. If we take one word and use different lettering we can see the difference (Fig. 6.4).

There are two different graphic aids available to help with lettering:

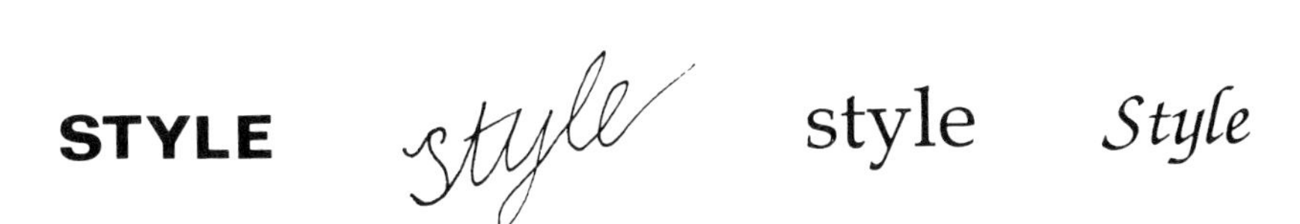

Fig. 6.4 By changing the type of lettering the same word can convey different meanings.

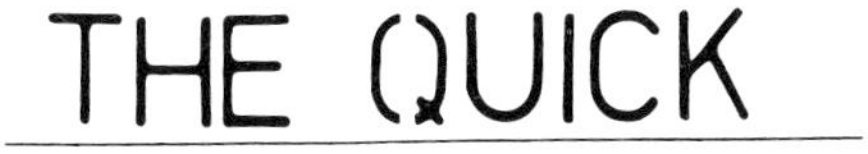

THE QUICK

Fig. 6.5 Stencil.

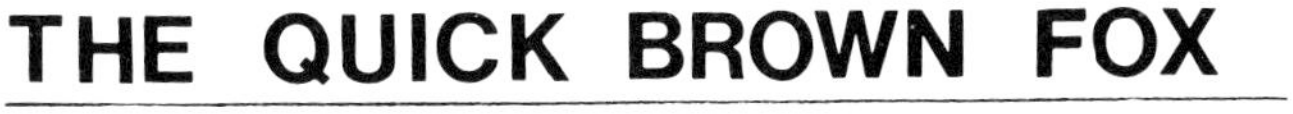

THE QUICK BROWN FOX

Fig. 6.6 Letraset.

(1) *Stencils.* These can be drawn onto a sheet of paper (Fig. 6.5). Remember to match the guideline underneath the letters to the one on your paper, so the word will be straight. Enlarge the result on a photocopier to the required size.
(2) *Letraset.* This is a transfer sheet of the complete alphabet and numbers, usually in black. You lay the transfer over your paper or card and rub it off onto it (Fig. 6.6). Again, remember to use a guideline so that all the letters sit on the same line. You can then enlarge them on a photocopier to the required size. Letraset is an extremely expensive way of working in time and materials.

A basic form of lettering can be carefully done without too much effort and cost, with good results, just by following a few golden rules.

(1) Make sure that the lettering you use is consistent and all in the same typeface.
(2) Always use a pencil first to draft the notice.
(3) Always use a ruler to calculate straight lines and spaces. Never attempt it free-hand.
(4) Always use guidelines.
(5) Always use reasonable quality thick paper or card.
(6) If you have a large area to colour then mask the edges with masking tape so they end up straight.

Figure 6.7 illustrates a simple method of lettering in bold capitals, with variations on the use of upper and lower cases (capitals and small letters), and a three-dimensional effect. Figure 6.8 illustrates the method of ‘free

SALON

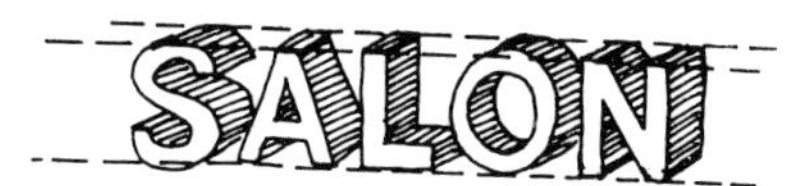

salon

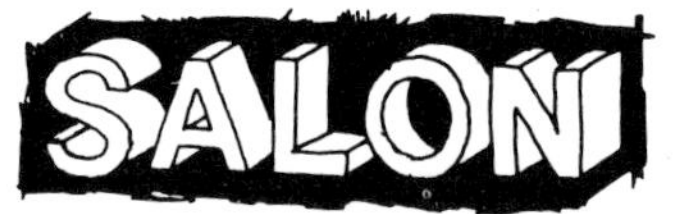

Fig. 6.7 Variations in lettering.

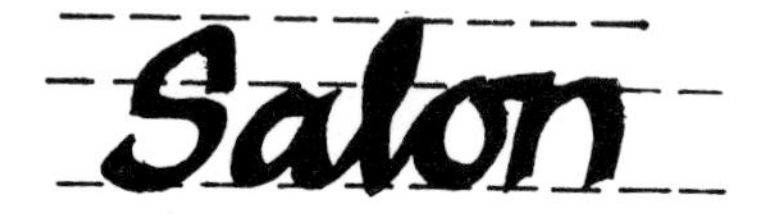

Fig. 6.8 Free handwriting using guidelines.

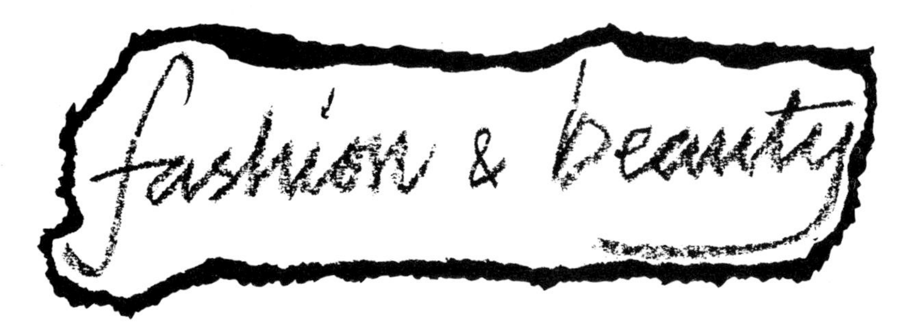

Fig. 6.9 Textural effect created by using a crayon.

handwriting' lettering. There are, of course, many more variations on lettering. You only have to look at any magazine or advertisement to see that. Also, the choice of drawing tool can give different effects. A currently popular technique, particularly used in magazines, is the use of crayon to give a textural effect when copied (Fig. 6.9). The choice of lettering is obviously yours but just remember, if it is your first attempt, to stick to something simple.

6.3 SALON ADVERTISING

Another use of advertising is of course promoting the actual salon, and the services it offers to the public. This can be done in various ways:

Salon cards. These should be freely available at the reception area and given out to clients, especially prospective clients who have just come in to make enquiries.

The cards should be clear and easy to read and contain only relevant information, such as the salon name, address and telephone number. A design, logo or motif can be added to give identity and a personal touch.

Salon 'menus' including services and prices (Fig. 6.10). These can be used as an alternative to salon cards and should also be readily available at the reception area. They can be excellent material for publicising the salon, as they give a professional touch and can be visually pleasing, which can encourage trade. They can be designed easily enough and printed. Again the more you have printed the cheaper the unit cost. Also, black and white can present quite a striking contrast and much cheaper to print than colour.

Salon advertising leaflets (Fig. 6.11). These can be produced by the salon with minimal office skills. Type a short text on a typewriter or, if possible, on a word processor, or if neither of these are available then write it by hand, neatly (observing the rules of lettering). This can then be pasted up on a sheet of paper accompanied with a design or simple line illustration. A variety of pre-drawn designs and images specifically for poster work is now available in many stationery shops, which can be helpful if you do not feel confident to do your own. The master copy can be photocopied or printed (depending on the quantity you want; it usually works out that the more you have the cheaper the unit cost) and hand-delivered through doors in your area to promote your salon or offer specific services.

Salon bags. Small paper bags with the salon name printed on them can be made without too much expense. These have a practical use and are a good investment if you sell your own products.

The media. Most areas have one or more free circular newspapers that would readily oblige if you contacted them to place an advertisement promoting your salon or services for a small fee. National newspapers and magazines on the other hand are extremely expensive, and there is no guaranteed return on your initial outlay.

Trade magazines of hairdressing and beauty will also charge a great deal to place an advertisement, although another way round is to send them, whenever possible, a selection of quality photographs of styles produced in your salon. They will sometimes feature them, and this is the best advertisement to promote your salon nationwide. Local radio stations will allow a small amount of air space, but again for a substantial cost, and of

THE SALON

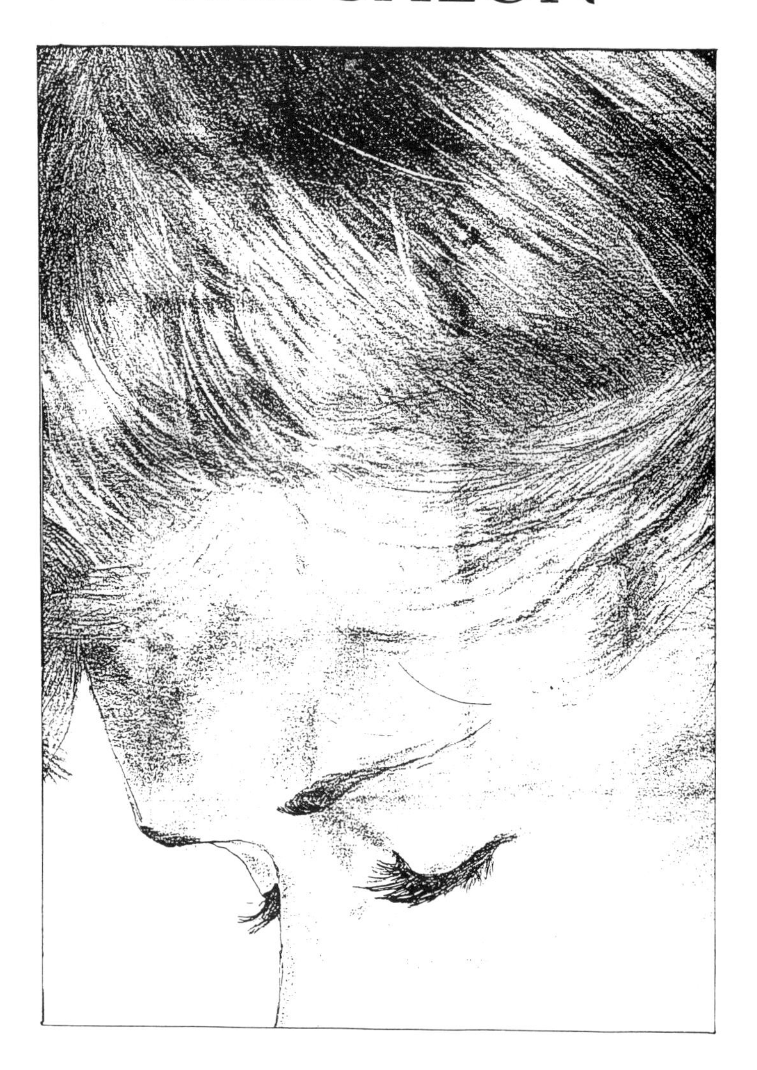

HAIR AND BEAUTY CENTRE

Fig. 6.10 Example of a salon 'menu' including services and prices.

HAIR AND BEAUTY AT THE SALON

HAIRDRESSING SERVICES

Wet Cut ....
Cut and Blow Dry ....
Restyle and Blow Dry ....
Wash and Blow Dry ....
Shampoo and Set ....

Perm ....
Root Perm ....
Molton Browners ....
Afro Curly Perm ....
Regrowth ....
Colour Tint ....
Regrowth ....
Semi-Permanent ....

Bleach ....
Roots ....
Highlights ....
Lowlights ....

Conditioning Treatments ....from

Relaxer ....
Regrowth ....

BEAUTY TREATMENTS

Facials ....from
Massage ....
Eyebrow Shape ....
Eyelash Tint ....
Manicure ....
Pedicure ....
Basic Make-up ....
Bridal Make-up ....
Party Make-up ....

THE SALON
99 The Street
Dulwich
S.E. 22

Tel: 071 111 1111

Open:-

Tuesday - Saturday 9.30 - 6.30

Late Night - Friday till 8.30

Special Price for Pensioners - Tuesdays

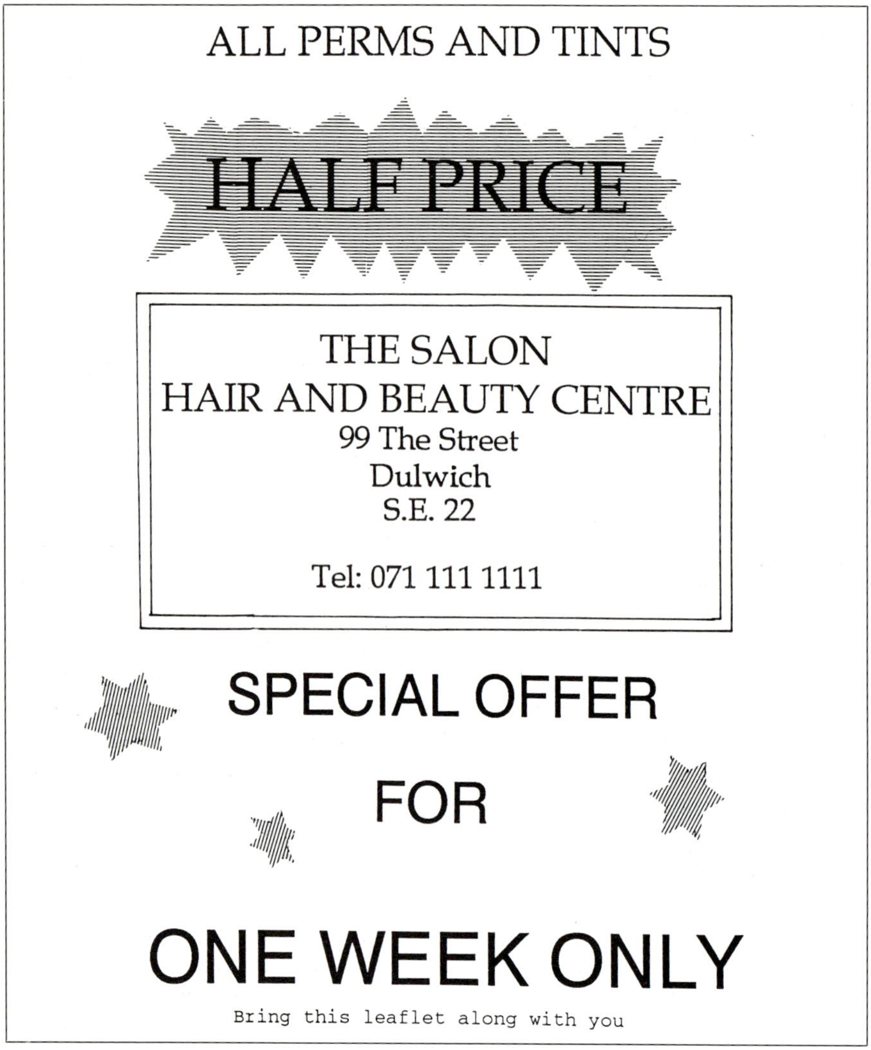

ALL PERMS AND TINTS

HALF PRICE

THE SALON
HAIR AND BEAUTY CENTRE
99 The Street
Dulwich
S.E. 22

Tel: 071 111 1111

SPECIAL OFFER

FOR

ONE WEEK ONLY

Bring this leaflet along with you

Fig. 6.11 Example of a salon leaflet advertising special offers.

course television is the pinnacle in advertising but you would need to remortgage your house to gain a couple of minutes of viewing time! Local television companies are becoming popular, so television advertising could become possible in the future. However, you must remember there would be much competition for advertising slots.

7

Photography

A good artist or designer will always keep records for reference and a hairdresser should follow the same practice. New styles that are created in the salon by the stylist or in college by the hairdressing trainee should be recorded as evidence of their artistic and technical ability, and indeed be used to illustrate their creative vocabulary. Once a newly created style has left the salon there is no record of it, so unless it is photographed it has gone forever.

Professional photographic sessions have to be tightly scheduled as time is money and delays can result in very expensive sessions. Professional photographers have to be pre-booked, which disallows any spontaneous creations that might evolve in the salon, or even good basic salon work. For these reasons it is important that hairdressers acquire basic photographic skills.

The camera is an extremely useful tool for the hairdresser and should be utilised to the full. A basic knowledge and understanding of how the camera works and its settings, appropriate lighting and composition are all that is needed to produce good professional-looking results. There is no mystique in photography. The camera is merely a mechanical eye recording a situation that you have created. It is within everyone's capability to take an adequate photograph, but you must be prepared to spend some time on preparation. It is preparation that will determine the quality of your results.

Having a personal portfolio of creative hair styles increases the confidence and credibility of the stylist and certainly instils a sense of confidence in the clientele. It also sets the right sort of creative atmosphere in the salon, encouraging good professional work.

Particularly good photographs could also be enlarged and used for advertising in the salon, or sent off to be featured in hairdressing, trade and beauty magazines, advertising the stylists' work and the salon nationwide. Many of the trade magazines have quite strict photographic requirements for prints that are submitted for publication. For instance, some prefer certain sizes of good quality black and white prints, while others might consider

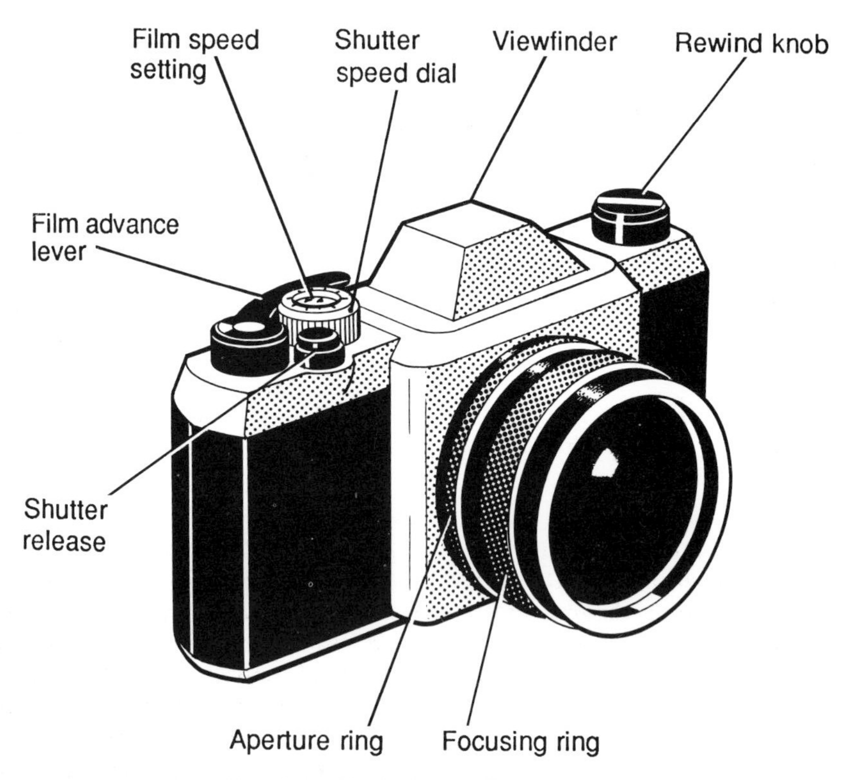

Fig. 7.1 Single lens reflex camera.

larger colour prints. It is worth finding out these requirements by telephoning the magazine and inquiring first, certainly before you start any photographing.

A currently successful use of photographs in promoting hair and make-up is the 'make-over', showing a photograph of the same model before and after styling. This could quite easily be adapted in the salon, and become an interesting advertising and promotions feature.

7.1 THE CAMERA (Fig. 7.1)

Basically the camera consists of a light-safe box, which houses your film. Attached to the front of it is a lens, which is adjusted in order to focus the image you wish to photograph onto your film. You look through a viewfinder in order to frame the subject you wish to record. When you press the shutter release button the film is momentarily exposed to light through the lens and the image is recorded on your film.

By far the most popular and versatile type of camera is the 35 mm single lens reflex (SLR). 35 mm indicates the size of film the camera takes. Single lens reflex means that, through the use of a mirror inside the camera body, you can look directly through the lens and see exactly the image that will be transposed onto your film. In other words you will see exactly what the camera will photograph.

There is a large range of interchangeable lenses available for this kind of camera, and consequently when different lenses are attached the effects will be instantly visible through the view-finder. The other advantage of this camera is that it is invariably fitted with an exposure meter. This can be used fully automatically or can have a manual override. The need for a manual override will become apparent later in this chapter.

There are two basic variables in the camera which control the exposure: one is the shutter speed and the other is the aperture or the F number.

(1) *Shutter speed.* This controls the length of time the shutter is held open for the exposure. The shutter speeds or stops, as they are called, are usually 1–2–4–8–15–30–60–125–250–500, and these represent fractions of a second. The larger the number the shorter the time during which light will reach the film. Each step up the sequence halves the amount of light reaching the film. The possibilities that this offers will now become obvious. Extremely fast shutter speeds will have the effect of freezing a fast-moving subject, rendering it motionless. Slower shutter speeds will make moving objects appear blurred. It is useful to note at this point that the camera should never be hand-held at speeds slower than 1/60th of a second because this can cause camera shake (the image will blur because of your hand movement). When shutter speeds slower than a 1/60th are required always use a tripod.

(2) *The aperture or F number.* Within the lens is fitted a diaphragm which can be opened or closed in order to let more or less light through the lens. The setting for the position of the diaphragm is known as the F number or stop. The F stops are F2, F2.8, F4, F5.6, F11, F16, F22. Each step up this sequence (as with the shutter speeds) halves the amount of light reaching the film.

The F number is used to control what is called 'the depth of field'. Usually in photographs not only the subject is in focus, but also objects in front and behind the subject. The extent to which objects are in focus in front of and behind your main image is known as depth of field. The higher the F number you use, the greater the distance in which all parts of the image on the photograph are in focus (from front to back). Conversely, the lower the F number you use the more shallow your depth of field will be. The advantage of this variable is not immediately apparent and need not concern us at this level. It will suffice to say that in a studio, by proper use of the F stops, selected features on the head may be placed in focus while foreground and background objects can be put out of focus.

As we now see, these two variables (shutter speeds and the F numbers) between them dictate the amount of light reaching the film. They need to be set correctly if the perfect exposure is to be achieved. As we have already mentioned, the fully automatic camera will do this for you: you merely need to focus the camera and take the picture. The advantage of a manual override in the camera means that you are in control of these two variables and can create specific effects.

7.2 FILM

There is a vast range of film on the market. It falls into three basic categories:

(1) Black and white.
(2) Colour negative for prints.
(3) Colour slides (or 'transparencies').

Colour films are produced specifically for either daylight work or studio work. All films have an ASA or DIN number. Photographers refer to this as the 'speed' of the film because it rates the speed with which the film reacts to light or in other words how sensitive the film is to light. The most common range of films available falls between 100 ASA (slow) and 400 ASA (fast), although they do come slower or faster than this. A film for use in average daylight would be 200 ASA. For indoor work without artificial light it is possible to use 400 ASA. Ideally if you are taking studio photographs you should use a slower film, with the aid of artifical light sources.

Remember, if you are using a 35 mm SLR camera you must set the camera to the corresponding speed of your film, in order for the meter in your camera to give the correct reading. This setting is usually found incorporated in the shutter speed dial.

Avoid wherever possible using a flash, because this creates a single frontal light source which tends to flatten the image of the subject. It can also create peculiar shadows, startle the sitters and reflect in their eyes.

7.3 LIGHTING

In the absence of proper studio facilities and lighting, makeshift situations can be created. Large windows are a source of abundant daylight. By sitting your subject next to the window and using white paper or sheets to reflect the light surprising results can be obtained (Fig. 7.2). More dramatic lighting can be created by using table lamps or spot lamps, although care must be taken that undesirable shadows are not cast. Also take into consideration if you are using colour film that most domestic lighting (tungsten) is of a warm orange hue and this will have a dramatic effect on the make-up and hair colour of the subject. If available use fluorescent lighting as this will give an effect closer to daylight. If you can, allow enough film for a certain degree of experimentation. Take the same shot using different exposure settings, i.e. over-expose and under-expose, and remember that if you have a built-in light meter your camera will be assessing the light value of the whole composition

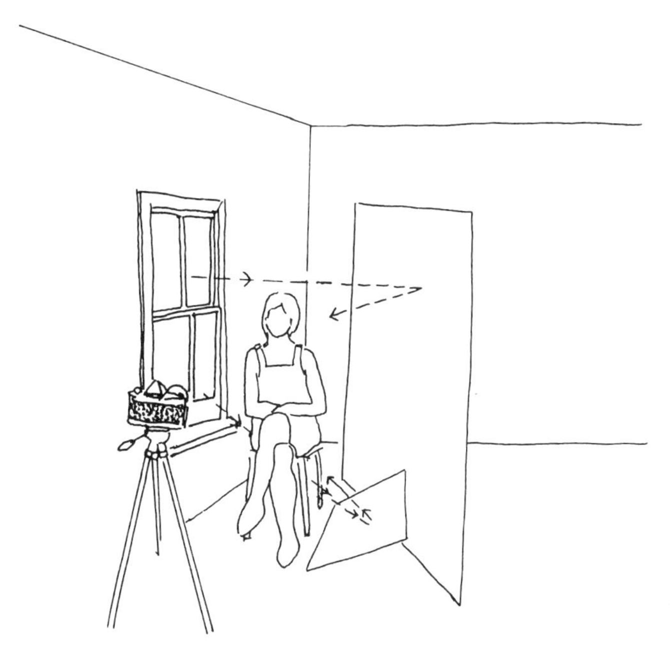

Fig. 7.2 Maximise light by using white surfaces or sheets to reflect it back onto the subject.

and not just your subject. It is only through experience that you can begin to predict the results.

7.4 COMPOSITION

The composition of your photograph must be considered from the very beginning, as soon as you look through the view-finder. Make sure that the object you wish to draw attention to is properly focused. Also balance and proportion are extremely important.

Place the subject in the centre of the photograph with enough space around it in order for it not to appear cramped on the one hand or lost in a void on the other (Fig. 7.4).

The need for balance and proportion applies not only to the subject and background, but also to the use of light and shade, and, if colour is used, to the primary and complementary colours within the composition. Contrasting lighting can produce dramatic or theatrical effects. You can use this to your advantage if you wish to highlight particular features.

When people are being photographed, a relaxed and spontaneous pose will give a more natural result. The sitter can be encouraged to smile or talk in order to break down any self-consciousness that may exist. Another alternative is to try a dummy run with an empty camera before you put the film in.

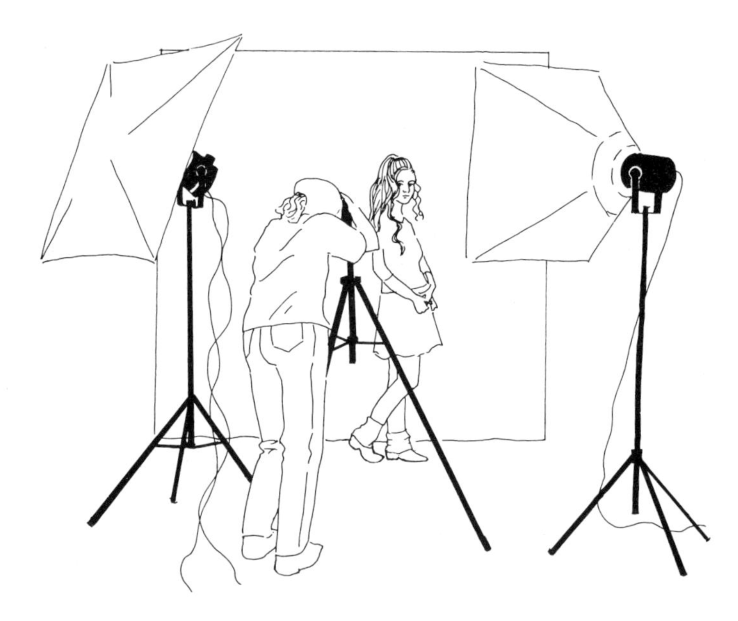

Fig. 7.3 Simple studio set-up – reflectors on the lights give a softer effect.

It is important to note that you should always pay as much attention to the background as you do to the subject. The background will enhance and make the most of your subject; use it to your advantage. Even props and a contrived setting can be introduced in order to create the right atmosphere which will enrich your composition. Always remember, when people look at your photographs the centre of attention should be dictated by you. Therefore remove all distracting elements so that the attention may be focused where you want it. If in doubt keep the backgrounds plain and simple.

7.5 MAKE-UP AND EFFECTS

It is important to make the most of your hard work and record your creative hair styles whether for your own reference, a portfolio or advertising photographs. You must make sure all the elements in the photograph blend together so that the hair and make-up complement one another. For instance, if you wish to record a good hair style you have created, it would make the photograph 100 per cent better to make sure the client's face is suitably made up. If you are using colour film then make sure the colours you use complement and that the picture is colour-balanced.

The look of the photograph can dictate the overall impression, so it is important to decide what image you are aiming for and make sure it comes across clearly. If the hair style is, for instance, aiming towards a soft, quieter image then make sure that the make-up is light and consists of paler tones,

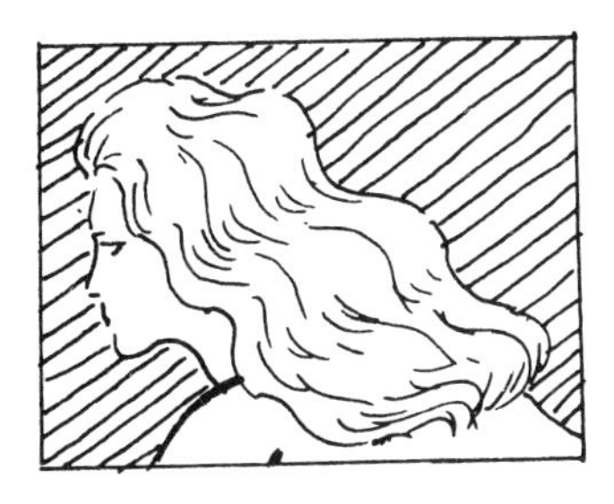

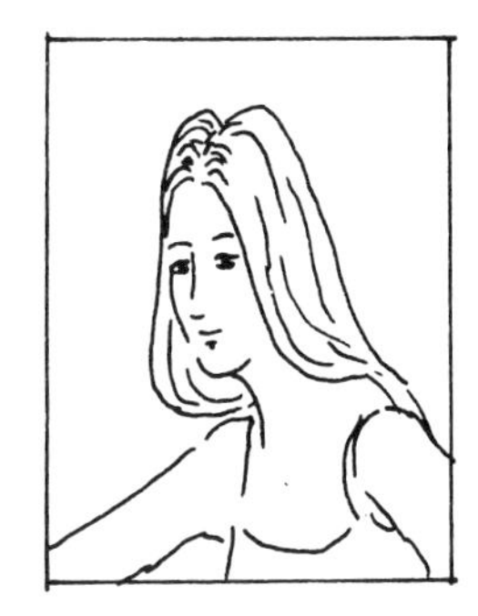

Fig. 7.4 Placing subject to create evenly balanced composition.

and that the background and lighting blend in with the image created by the soft pastel colours. On the other hand if your intentions are more geared towards creating a fashion image, then the model should have make-up that is more vibrant in colour and with enough contrast to accentuate the eyes, bone-structure and lips. The lighting should also be chosen to enhance contrast, and the background could be more lively. It would be wonderful if all hairdressers were in a financial position that allowed them to employ a professional make-up artist, but that is not always the case and quite honestly you do not need to have fantastic skills in applying make-up. Just a little knowledge of what, how and where will enable you to achieve the right effect and enrich your photographs.

The aim of using make-up is basically to enhance the features, add colour and to balance the face with the use of highlighting and shading. Different colour choices can create different effects; for instance, colours that complement the model's own warm skin tones will heighten the warmth, whereas colours that contrast with the skin tones will give a sharper or stark appearance.

It is important to remember that colour can react quite differently on different coloured skin tones; for instance, a blue eye-shadow can look extremely subtle on a fair skin, yet vibrant on a black skin.

The choice of make-up is also important. The most important feature when choosing is to get a good colour range in foundations, eye-shadows, pencils, and lipsticks, using as many different brands as need be. The quality of make-up is not so important, unless the model needs to keep it on for any extended length of time or if the make-up leans more towards the theatrical, when special make-up needs to be applied. It would be a worthwhile investment for the salon to buy a good range of make-up for photographic and promotional use.

Face. Apply a foundation that matches the model's skin tone, and apply it, preferably with a make-up sponge, evenly over the face, not forgetting to blend it down into the neck so a line does not show around the jaw. A good tip is to skim gently over the whole face and neck with a piece of dampened cotton wool after applying foundation as this will ensure a smooth blend.

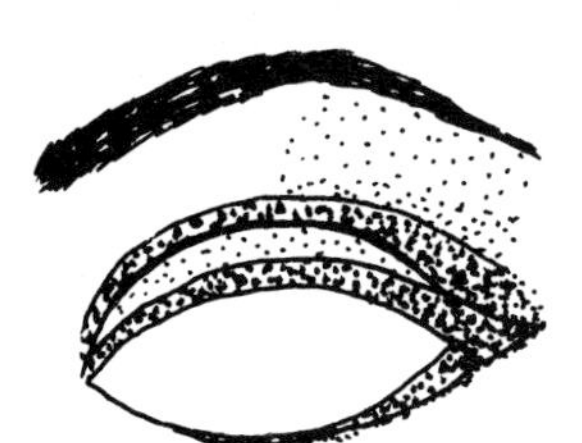

Fig. 7.5 Application of eye make-up.

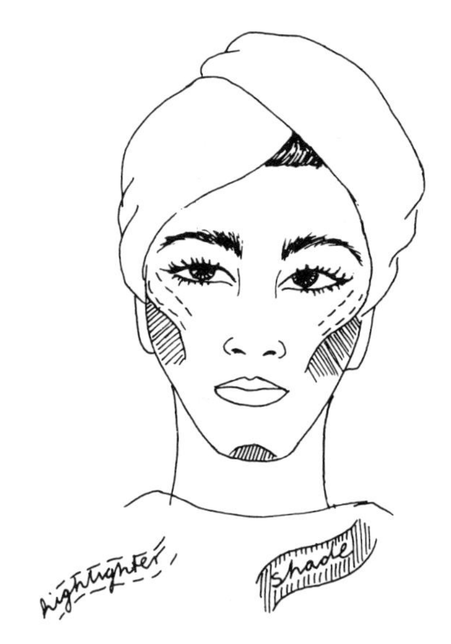

Fig. 7.6 Basic use of highlighter and shade on the face for photographic work, to emphasise the bone structure.

Afterwards, fix the foundation with a translucent powder as this will make a good even basis for applying make-up and it will also stop any unwanted shining.

Eyes. Apply eye-shadows by using a brush and starting with the lighter colours first. The general aim is to lengthen the eye by exaggerating the outer corners. This can be achieved by applying a lighter eye-shadow on the upper lid and below the eyebrow and then applying a darker shadow to outline the eye. For a stronger effect an eyeliner pencil can also be used, but use brown as black will appear too heavy. The eye can be further accentuated by applying a darker eye-shadow along the eye socket line. Lastly, apply some mascara to the upper and lower lashes (Fig. 7.5).

Eyebrows. These are best left natural, although they might need tidying and lengthening; in this case use an eye pencil, but again, not black.

Cheeks. The aim of shading (Fig. 7.6) is to emphasise the bone structure, so apply blusher underneath the check bones using a brush. If your model sucks in her cheeks this will indicate where to put the blusher, but be careful not to extend it too far into the face or she will look like a doll.

Blusher can also be applied to the tip of the nose to make it appear shorter. The forehead can be made to appear narrower by shading either side at the temples. The chin can be shortened by applying a little blusher at the base and slightly under the chin. Wherever you use blusher, make sure it is blended well!

Lips. It is easy and most hygienic to use a brush to apply lipstick if possible. First outline the lips with a lip pencil that is slightly darker than the lipstick you intend to use, then apply the lipstick evenly. Avoid using red unless you intend a harsh result as it will appear black on black and white prints. If you want a sensuous effect then apply lip gloss over the top.

7.6 PERSONAL PORTFOLIO

Hairdressers should from an early point in their careers, get into the habit of collecting good quality photographs of their work. From the time of training at college or in the salon, whenever they are pleased with a style they have produced they should record it so that when they are fully accomplished stylists it will have become second nature to record good or fashionable styles or more creative work. Keeping a portfolio of your own work is essential to any designer, as it illustrates very clearly the variation of your work, the versatility of your skills, the potential of your creative ability and your degree of professionalism.

There are different types of portfolios available to buy depending on how much you are willing to spend. They range from a simple A4 photograph album available from most stationery shops to more plush professional-looking A3 or A4 zip portfolios available from most art shops. Whichever type you choose, it is the contents and presentation of the work in the end that is more important. The portfolio should include quality photographs that portray a good range of styles, demonstrating skills on short, medium and long hair, also on different textures, coarse, fine etc., and a variety of hair types, straight, curly, thin, thick, etc. If possible include hair styles on different racial types, e.g. European, Afro, Oriental etc. The styles should show a good mastery of techniques: cutting, perming, blow-drying, long hair, setting, plaiting etc. This will demonstrate your good basic hairdressing skills.

Work leaning towards the creative can be more specialised, such as the use of different colouring techniques demonstrating more of an imaginative approach to the subject. High fashion work or innovative ideas will reflect your creative potential. Another good feature is to include a case study on a model. First, analyse all the features influencing the model's style choice: face shape, facial and body features, colour, dress, personality, image, lifestyle, etc. and then offer a range of suitable hair styles. Perhaps include the styles she would be best to avoid too. Also 'make-overs' look effective, showing a model before and after styling, perhaps with and without make-up.

A good portfolio is a useful asset when applying for a job, or in particular when wanting to move on to other areas of work, such as television, film, or magazines. It will enhance your career prospects, but you must remember to keep it updated. A good portfolio that stopped five years ago loses its impact.

Another interesting portfolio idea that will show an imaginative and creative mind is to keep a portfolio of personal interest and ideas. This, like an artist's sketch-book, reveals the creative potential. Interesting advertisements, magazine cuttings of current fashion trends, popular images or favourite personalities, anything really that is of interest to the hairdresser, can be included. The presentation for this portfolio can apply a freer approach. Collage is usually the most effective: a juxtaposition of images overlapping and arranged in an interesting way. This type of personal portfolio will reinforce the portfolio of your work when furthering your career.

8

The Total Look

Style is not a new word in fashion: different fashion styles have been with us for a very long time. Up until the 1960s and 1970s fashion designers created complete fashion styles including every detail so that one hair style or hat, for instance, was always worn with a particular dress to produce the style the fashion designer intended. Sometimes the personal styles of film stars or pop idols were emulated, but whatever the actual source, the inspiration nearly always came from above and was copied by ordinary people as closely as they could.

A new force has emerged in the fashion world over the last fifteen to twenty years that has broken the hold of this hierarchical system. This is the emergence of 'street fashion', which has recognised the potential of innovative youth to choose whatever combinations of fashions they think appropriate to project their own images. This new trend blends together all the different fashion areas (hair, cosmetics, clothes, accessories) in countless ways to create exciting new images. The emphasis is on the image created rather than on the clothes alone, and this is why the new movement has been described as 'fashion styling' or sometimes 'image making'.

This new attitude to fashion has forced the once various fashion industries closer together and compelled them to work in co-operation in order to survive in an ever changing and highly competitive field. Cosmetics and hair products are now promoted by marrying them to an image or look. Whether the image is soft, sultry or sophisticated, it is this that is sold not the actual product.

There is now a new type of designer who recognises the potential of combining the three main areas of fashion (clothes, hair styles and make-up), and is aware of the variety of images that can be created. These new designers are known as 'stylists'. They are fully equipped with the skills to produce different 'total look' images for promotions, photographs, film or television. There are now some courses in fashion styling provided in further and higher education colleges.

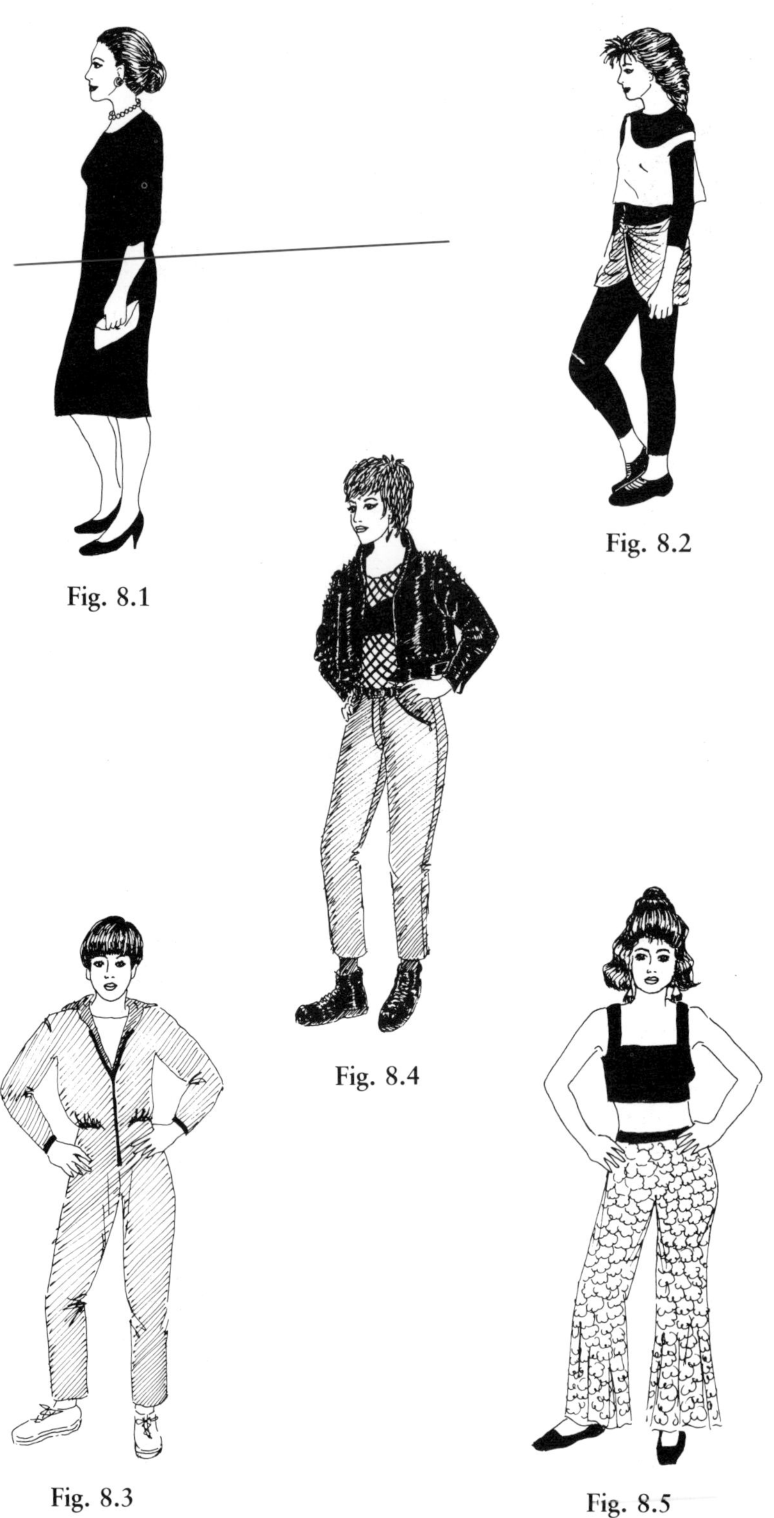

Fig. 8.1

Fig. 8.2

Fig. 8.4

Fig. 8.3

Fig. 8.5

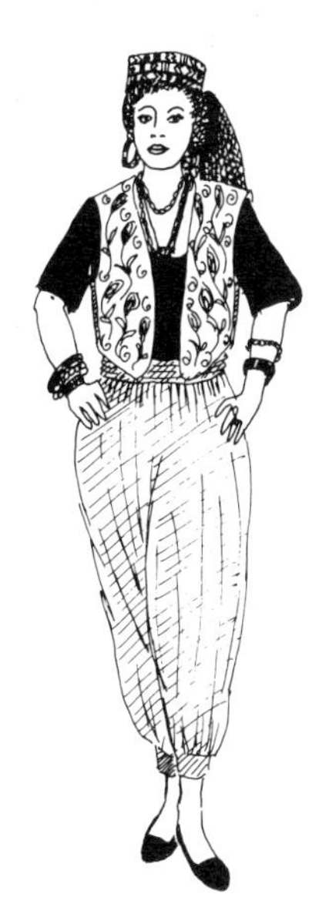

Fig. 8.6

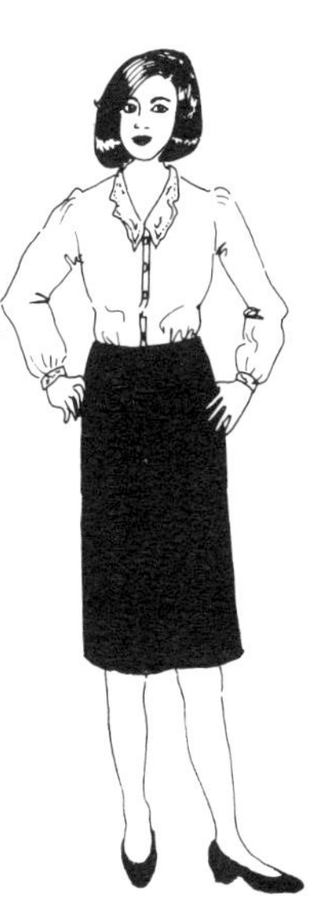

Fig. 8.7

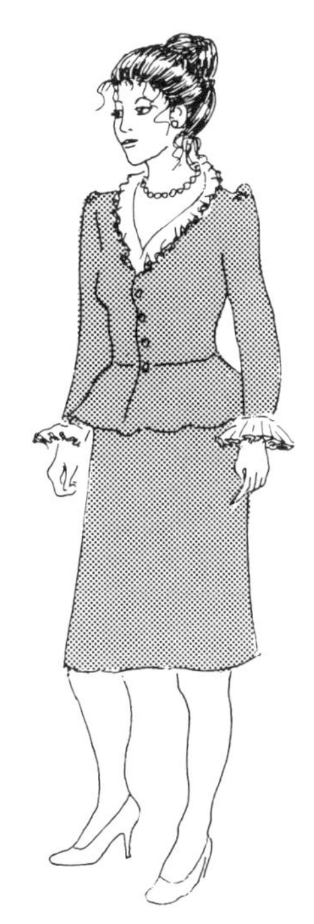

Fig. 8.9

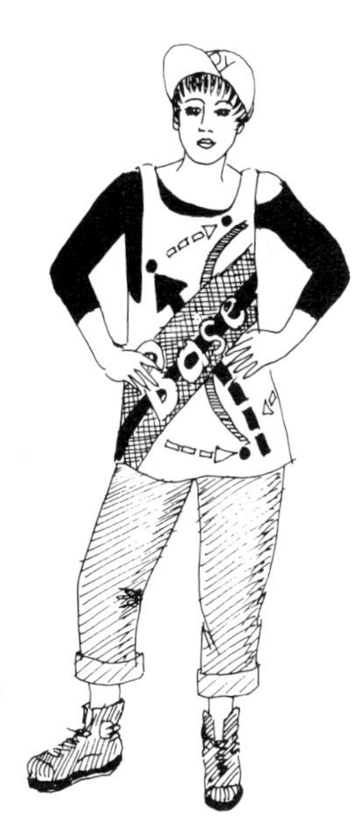

Fig. 8.8

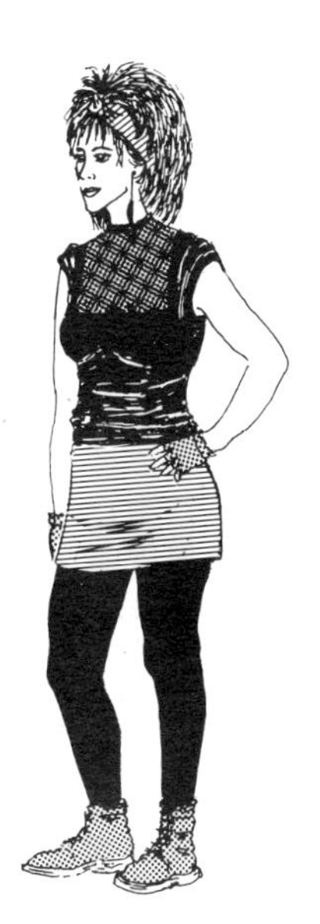

Fig. 8.10

Hairdressers make an essential contribution to fashion styling and the creation of the total look because the styles they create help to determine the image the client projects. They should not only have the skills and enthusiasm to adapt readily to new ideas that evolve and become fashionable, but they should also be innovators themselves. They should be able to create new fashion ideas themselves and to develop the new techniques required to realise their ideas in practice.

It is important then that hairdressers should firstly recognise that different images exist, that they should be able to identify them, and that they should have some idea of the hair styles and hair accessories that enhance them. Hairdressers should keep a close eye on different fashion magazines that represent different sections of the public, or certainly different age groups. Some examples of magazines to watch are: *Vogue*, *Elle*, *Cosmopolitan*, *Harpers and Queen*, *Looks*, *Just 17*, *The Face*, and *Smash Hits*. Fashion and media programmes on the television are also useful, and if you live in a big town or city you can watch the various images that exist on the streets. Acknowledgement of what is around you will help in the process of being able to identify different looks and it could also act as an inspirational springboard for creating new ideas.

Categorising images can be a difficult task. Figs 8.1–8.10 show some examples of the images that are around:

- fashionable
- sophisticated
- hippy
- conservative
- feminine
- sporty
- hard
- punk
- ethnic
- tomboy

Can you match the image to each picture?

Total looks or fashion images, of course, are not solely inspired by creating new ideas from within our own fashion world. Like every other creative field, fashion takes its inspiration from all different aspects of life, and particularly from different cultures and the world around us. Different ethnic looks have been incorporated successfully with Western fashions over the last twenty to thirty years. Designers take a particular feature and combine it with their own ideas to produce a new trend or style. This is an extremely fruitful move by designers because in this melting pot of ideas many new combinations of styles can emerge. Another new trend to emerge, not so deliberate and certainly not designed, is a sort of cultural street fashion. This happens when ethnic minorities in a country continue to wear their traditional dress, but adapt it to their new circumstances. For instance silk saris are worn here in Britain with woolly cardigans or thick anoraks to compensate for the cool climate.

Let us take a look at some different ethnic looks that are around today and have avoided too much Western intervention. Looking at them in their purity, so to speak, clearly illustrates the individuality of each different country and culture.

8.1 DIFFERENT LOOKS FROM AROUND THE WORLD

Africa

Within Africa itself racial characteristics vary enormously from the tone of the skin to the height and even body shapes of people in different regions. Skin tone, for instance, is light in northern African countries such as Morocco, and blue/black in certain tribes south of the Sahara desert. Although fabric designs, particularly patterns and colours can also vary dramatically from region to region the traditional costumes or most popular forms of dress in Africa basically fall into three categories (Figs 8.11 and 8.12).

(1) The wrapper

The wrapper is a length of material, usually cotton, that is worn around the body and across the breast falling to mid-calf or ankle length. A separate length of the same material, called a stole, is worn over the shoulder, hanging down onto the body. The colours are usually quite bright.

The most popular headwear seems to be the head tie, which consists of a separate piece of the same material used to wrap around the head and tied. The variations in how this cloth is tied seem endless. The tie and how it is worn is supposed to express the mood of the wearer.

(2) The up and down

The up and down is usually made from thin cotton, brightly dyed and usually designed with bold patterns. This garment is more fitted to the body than the wrapper, accentuating the female shape more. It has a separate top worn with an ankle-length skirt. This garment again is usually worn with some form of head tie, usually in the same material.

(3) The kaftan

The kaftan is a loose-flowing robe that can be made either of light-weight cotton or a finer material such as silk. It is popular particularly in regions where there is a strong Muslim influence.

The kaftan is not so colourful and bold in design as the wrapper and the up and down. It is usually made of a plainer material and decorated with an embroidered border design and yoke. The kaftan was adopted by the black Americans in the 1960s and 70s as a symbol of black power along with the Afro hair style. It is often worn with a variety of headwear, in particular a fez-style of hat.

India

Indian fashions have a distinct look, combining fine fabrics with articulate designs. An important feature of the dress is the addition of jewellery such as

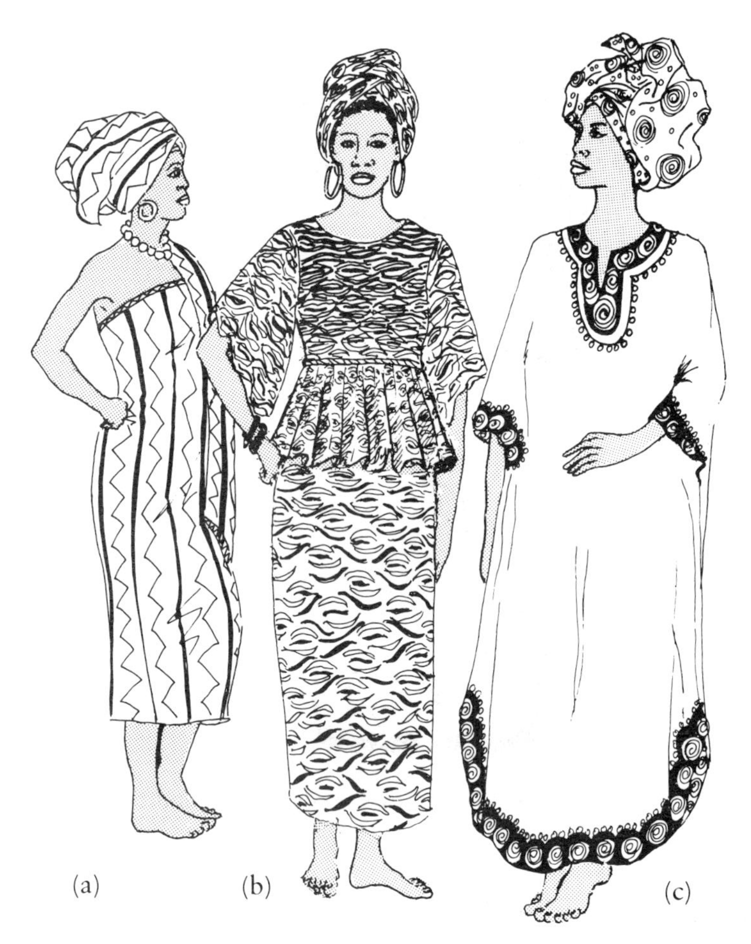

Fig. 8.11 The three main categories of traditional African costumes: (a) wrapper; (b) up and down; (c) kaftan.

bracelets and rings. Nose ornaments are customary. Other customary features of Indian culture are the painted circle worn in the middle of the forehead distinguishing caste and the painting with henna of women's hands and feet, which is believed to have a magical effect on marriage. There is a wide variety of fabric designs, patterns and colours, but basically there are four main garments worn (Fig. 8.13).

(1) The sari

The sari is probably the most recognised traditional Indian costume, and must surely be the most elegant. It is a length of material, usually silk (although other cheaper materials are worn), which is basically wrapped around the body. It is worn with a blouse. The Hindu religion requires modesty in women, particularly married women, so the material is drawn up to cover the head when in public.

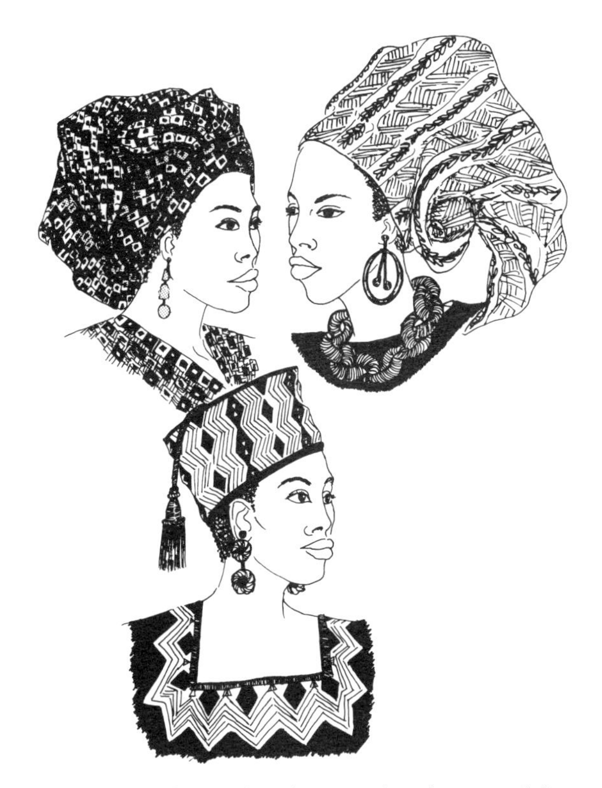

Fig. 8.12 African headwear – head ties and fez.

(2) The ghagra

The ghagra consists of a long pleated fine cotton skirt reaching down to the ankles. It is worn with a tight-fitted cotton or silk blouse called a choli. A scarf or orhna, which is a separate length of material, is worn draped over the head and shoulders and is sometimes used as a veil to cover the face.

(3) The salwar

Muslim religion plays a strong part in the popularity of this garment. It consists of loose-fitting trousers, usually made of silk, which are gathered at the foot by a sort of cuff. These are worn with a long tunic, also in silk, reaching down to mid-thigh, called a kameez. It is also worn with a scarf covering the head, or draped across the shoulders.

(4) The sarong

The sarong is a product of Western influence, although it is still worn in rural parts of India. It is basically a length of cotton or silk wrapped around the body across the breasts and reaching down to calf-length. It is usually much bolder in design, probably because of the Western influence.

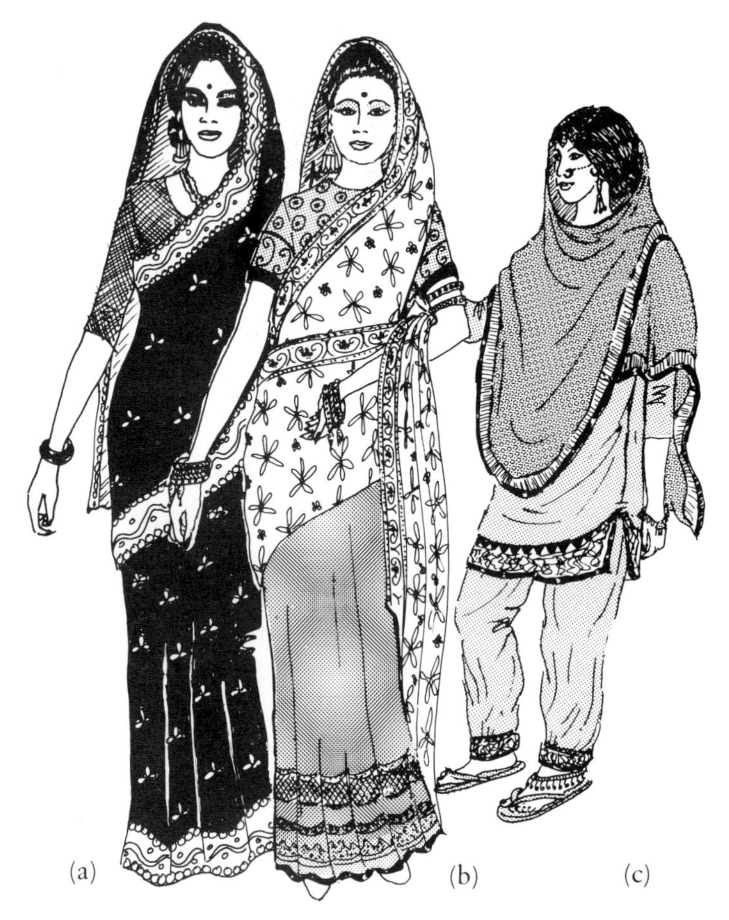

Fig. 8.13 Indian fashions: (a) sari; (b) ghagra; (c) salwar.

South America

The costume of South American countries such as Brazil and Peru has been subject to outside influence ever since the arrival of the Spanish explorers in the 16th century. Inca civilisation was wiped out by the Europeans, and, later still, European features were taken up, such as the wearing of bowler hats by women in Bolivia, a trend adopted from British workmen who built the railway there. However, a distinctive South American look has emerged and survived through all these influences (Fig. 8.14).

The clothes and fabrics are very colourful, with beautifully woven shawls and small boleros. The costume usually consists of huge skirts called polleras, which are made of heavy cotton and reach down to mid-calf. These are worn with a blouse and sometimes a brightly woven or printed waistcoat. On top of this might be a finely woven blanket worn over the shoulders as a sort of poncho, or just draped over one shoulder. Women also wear an aguayo,

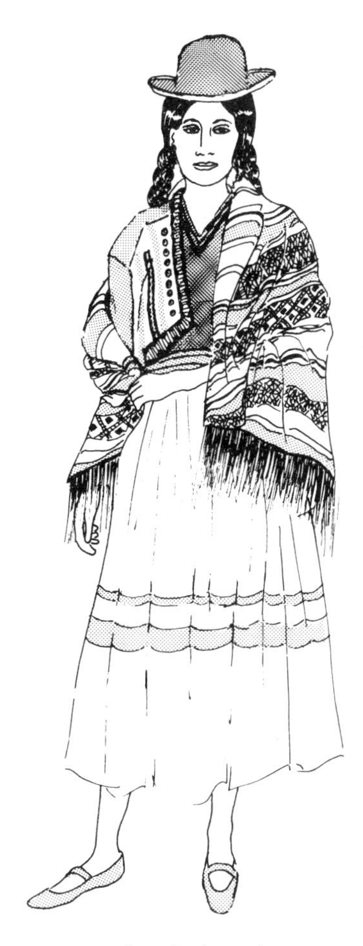

Fig. 8.14 South American costume.

which is a striped cotton shawl, wrapped around the body and used to carry a baby at the back.

Most women wear their hair in two hanging plaits, and some cover the head with a tied scarf, but more often than not they will wear a hat.

Japan

Traditional Japanese costume (Fig. 8.15) is not simply a garment, but more of a spiritual experience. The kimono is designed, like most things in Japanese culture, to promote discipline. The garment straightens the posture and restricts excessive movement. How the kimono looks on a woman is supposed to reveal her inner qualities; it is supposed to reflect the beauty of the spirit and character.

Kimono translated means thing (*mono*) wear (*ki*), and although it is the

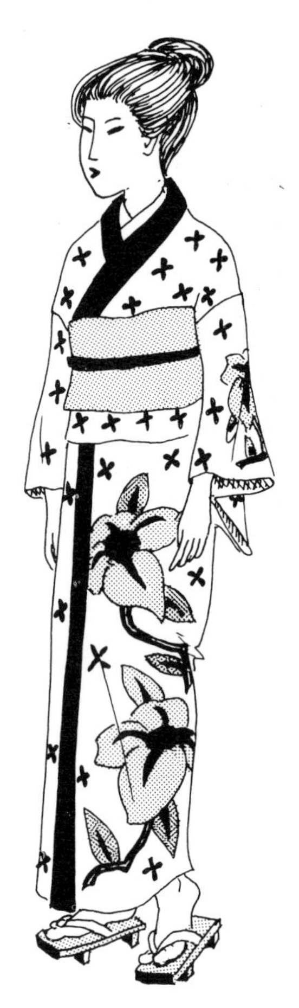

Fig. 8.15 Kimono.

traditional Japanese dress, today it is really only used for ceremonial costume about two or three times a year. Western style of dress, after about the mid-19th century, influenced the traditional Japanese style of dress (more so for men than for women), but then in 1945 after the Second World War, due to wartime shortages, the wearing of the kimono amongst Japanese women practically ceased. Recently there seems to have been a positive move to re-instate the kimono as traditional dress and encourage more women to wear it more often. The kimono can be made of silk, cotton, linen or even wool, although synthetic fabric mixes have made it more affordable. The colours have to be harmonised. For instance, colours worn have to correspond to those of flowers and plants in season. Sometimes on top of the kimono women wear an obi, which is a sort of belt folded neatly at the back.

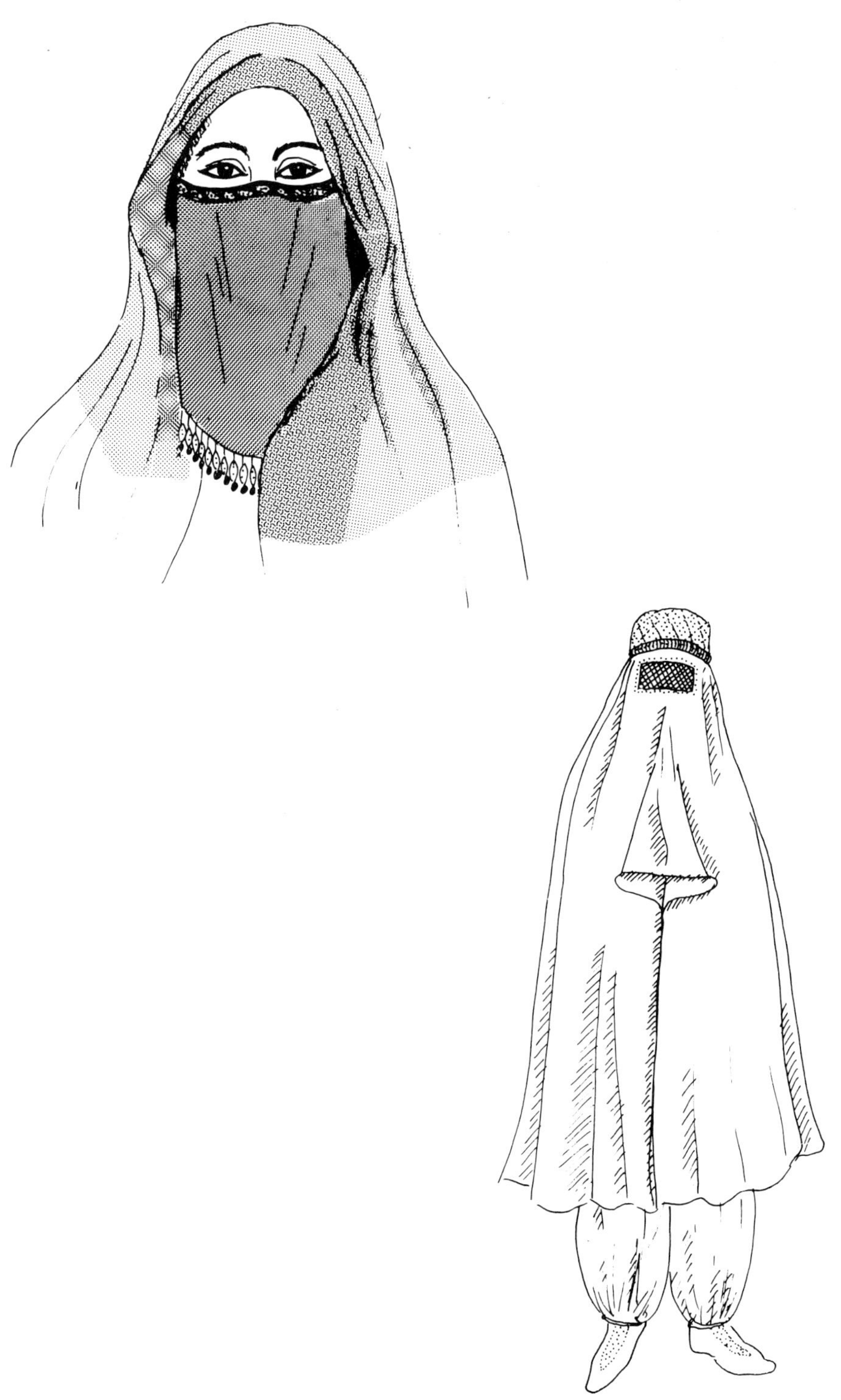

Fig. 8.16 Female Muslim costume and yashmak.

Arab countries

The Muslim religion is the strongest influence on Arab dress (Fig. 8.16). The religion demands that women cover their bodies and hair once they have reached puberty. Some Muslim cultures are more strict than others about this, forbidding any part of the body to be shown, so women wear loose-fitting trousers along with a burqa, a long enveloping headdress. The headdress has a fine grid of woven cloth inserted across the face area so the woman can see out, but no-one can see in. The costume is usually made of fine cotton or linen, and the colour is usually white or black. Other cultures are not so strict and the costume usually consists of women wearing loose-fitting gowns that reach down to the feet. The head is covered by a length of material draped also over the shoulders. The hair is always covered, and in some cases the yashmak (a thin veil which hides the bottom half of the face) is worn.

8.2 DEVELOPING THE TOTAL LOOK

This book has shown you the principles of design – how to use line and colour and apply the rules of balance and symmetry. It has also provided a mass of ideas in the different looks and fashions throughout history and across the world. These are the tools used by the stylist, and all that is needed apart from them are the inspiration and imagination of the individual designer to create new and exciting images.

It is an ideal opportunity when hairdressers are training to encourage these styling skills. It is important to develop a sense of awareness of the body as a whole, and of the hair and head as an integral part of the body. Exercises in designing whole images or a total look from a theme or idea from history or nature might result in slightly theatrical images, but they give valuable practice in seeing the image as a whole. This is an excellent starting-point and a good opportunity for trainees to be creative as well as demonstrating their technical skills.

Total look shows or demonstrations in colleges or private schools can offer the trainee this opportunity to research and create new ideas on live models. It can be a lot of fun for everyone too!

Index

art deco, 112–13
asymmetrical styles, 18–19

case study, 16
colour
  addition, 25
  co-ordination, 143
  cool, 29, 32
  depth of, 30
  discordant, 31
  expression, 33
  hair, 30–31
  harmonious, 31
  lighting, 24–5, 34
  monochromatic, 31
  neutralising, 28–32
  pigment, 25–6, 30
  primary, 26–8
  seasonal, 33
  secondary, 26–7
  shade charts, 30
  subtraction, 25
  symbolism, 33, 62, 90
  temperature, 146
  tone, 31–2
  warm, 29, 31
crown, 57
  double, 57

extensions, 76, 135

facial profile, 15, 47–8
four stem braid, 22–3

graduated cut, 6

hairlines
  cow's lick, 56–7
  nape, 56–7
  neck, 57
  receding, 56
  temples, 57
  widow's peak, 56–7
hair partings, 57–8
hair styles
  apollo knot, 106
  bob, 81–2, 125, 134–5
    French, 113–14
  bouffant, 122–3
  bowl crop, 84–5, 88
  Brutus cut, 102, 108
  chignon, 107–8
  cropped, 134–5
  Eton crop, 113–14
  garconne, 125
  gypsy cut, 129
  Marcel waving, 108
  orbis, 71
  page-boy, 118
  permanent waving, 117

plaiting, 22–3, 62, 65, 74, 76–7, 80, 126, 128, 135, 176
polled, 87
pompadour, 109, 111
ponytail, 120, 135
punk, 129–31, 134
Purdy cut, 129
shingle, 113–14
textured, 135
urchin cut, 120
Victorian bun, 107
wedge, 129
hair types, 7–11, 57–8
Afro hair, 7, 165
cut, 126
Asian hair, 8, 165
coarse hair, 11
curly hair, 11
European hair, 8, 165
fine hair, 10
Oriental hair, 8, 165
straight hair, 11
thick hair, 11
thin hair, 10
hats
bicorne, 106
boater, 108
bowler, 106, 174–5
chaperon, 82
cloche, 114
flat caps, 115
mob caps, 101
phrygian, 77
pinners, 101
taffeta pipkin, 91–2
tam-o-shanter, 106
tricorne, 97
trilby, 117
turban, 118–19
headdresses
African headties, 171, 173
atlifet, 91–2
barbette, 77, 80, 82–4
bonnet, 87
butterfly, 83
cache peigne, 107–8
chimney pot, 83–4
circlet, 81–2
coif, 77–8, 88
crespine, 80–82, 91
cushion, 81–2
Egyptian nems, 63
fillet, 77
fontange, 96
French hood, 86, 91
gable, 87
split, 87
gorget, 77
henin, 83–4, 87
horned, 83
Muslim burqa, 177–8
snood, 80, 91, 108, 118–19
steeple, 83–4
tower, 96
wimple, 77, 87
yashmak, 177–8
head shapes, 48–9

khol, 64–5, 73, 114

layered cut, 4
long, 6

one length cut, 6

pattern
block repeat, 18, 20
diamond repeat, 18, 20
half-drop repeat, 18, 20
positive and negative, 21–2
rotating shapes, 18, 20
photographs, 140, 157, 161, 165
make-up for, 162–5
punk, 129–31
Gothic, 130–32

salon
design, 142–3, 145–6
furnishings, 143–5
image, 138–9, 142
lighting, 34, 146
window display, 139–41
six strand plait, 22–3

street fashion, 126, 132–3, 167–70
stylists, 167

three strand plait, 21, 23

unisex
  fashions, 126
  hairdressing, 142

wigs, 62–3, 71, 88, 91, 106, 126
  Afro, 126
  double peaked, 97, 99
  full bottomed, 97, 102
  peri, 96
  queued, 102, 108